The House Physician's H

The House Physician's Handbook

C. Allan Birch
M.D., F.R.C.P.
Honorary Consulting Physician
Chase Farm Hospital, Enfield, Middlesex

S. J. Surtees
M.B., M.R.C.P.E., F.R.C.Path., D.T.M. & H
Consultant Chemical
Pathologist and Postgraduate
Clinical Tutor,
Eastbourne Health District,
East Sussex

Richard Wray
M.B., M.R.C.P.
Consultant Physician, Hastings Health District

FIFTH EDITION

CHURCHILL LIVINGSTONE
EDINBURGH LONDON AND NEW YORK 1980

CHURCHILL LIVINGSTONE
Medical Division of the Longman Group Limited

Distributed in the United States of America by
Churchill Livingstone Inc., 19 West 44th Street, New
York, N.Y. 10036, and by associated companies,
branches and representatives throughout the world.

First edition 1955
Second edition 1962
Third edition 1972
Fourth edition 1977
Fifth edition 1980

ISBN 0 443 02117 1

British Library Cataloguing in Publication Data
Birch, Charles Allan
  The House Physician's handbook. - 5th ed.
  1. Interns (Medicine) – Great Britain
  I. Title II. Surtees, S.J
  III. Wray, Richard
  616   RA972   79-40864

Printed in Hong Kong by
Wilture Enterprise (International) Co Ltd

Preface to the Fifth Edition

In this fifth edition the division into four chapters is retained but the work of revising them has been shared by three authors. We have been guided as before by what house physicians said they felt the book should include. We are grateful to many colleagues for helpful suggestions and particularly to Mr M. Bastable, F.I.M.L.S. Dr Donald McKendrick has kindly allowed us to use the table on the Policy for Infectious Diseases in General Wards from his chapter in the forthcoming eleventh edition of *Emergencies in Medical Practice*.

The table of diagnostic tests in chapter 3 now contains about 400 items arranged alphabetically with details of collection requirements, 'normal' values and comments on significance.

Cisternal puncture has been omitted as it is outside the province of the house physician. Since smallpox was officially declared eradicated in May, 1980 the technique of vaccination is omitted. Most values are given in traditional and SI units, the latter being stated first, but drug concentrations are still reported in mass units. The basic facts on the use of the subclavian vein for temporary cardiac pacing and for i.v. feeding are briefly stated since these procedures, after practical instruction, are within the competence of many house physicians.

We have always been watchful of the work of house physicians and hope that the information offered in this edition will help many future residents in their early years.

1980

C Allan Birch

J J Fulkes

Richard Wray.

Contents

1 General Information

2 Clinical procedures

3 The Medical Laboratory

4 Treatment

Introduction

Your resident post in hospital provides a great opportunity for you to learn about the continuing care of the patients under your charge. Make the most of this. Watch carefully day by day the course of illness and the effect of treatment. Learn all you can of the art of prognosis and of dealing with relatives.

Much of this book is about the technical procedures used in diagnosis and treatment but you should not regard your patients merely as interesting 'cases' on whom to use these techniques. They are human beings, many of them anxious, worried and full of doubts and fears. The picture each presents will be coloured by his emotional make-up. Always remember that you are treating patients and not diseases for as Trousseau said long ago, 'Il n'y a pas de maladies, il n'y que des malades.'

For all patients the best doctor is the one who can best inspire hope. In all your work therefore, do not forget the human touch.

''Tis the human touch in this world that counts,
    The touch of your hand on mine,
Which means far more to the fainting heart
    Than shelter and bread and wine,
For shelter is gone when the night is o'er,
    And bread lasts only a day,
But the touch of the hand and the sound of the voice
    Sing on in the soul alway.'

Spencer Michael Free 1856–1938
M.D. Johns Hopkins 1880

1

General information

ON ARRIVAL

1. Try to meet your predecessor before he leaves and learn from him any peculiarities of the job.

2. Fairly soon after arrival make yourself familiar with the administrative arrangements of the Laboratory, the X-ray Department, the Pharmacy, the Records Department and the Social Worker's Office. Many hospitals give new residents a copy of the standing orders and a description of their job.

3. Make sure that you are a member of a Medical Defence Society and that your subscription is not in arrears. (Most Area Health Authorities make this a condition of employment.)

4. Find out exactly where drugs and instruments for emergencies are kept. If there is an Emergency Cupboard you should know what is in it and where the key is kept.

ON DEPARTURE

1. Complete and return all outstanding case notes.

2. Return all library books and keys.

3. Ask your chief for a testimonial and, if yours was a preregistration post, a certificate of satisfactory service.

GENERAL ADVICE

1. Don't put a practitioner through a *viva voce* when he requests a bed for his patient. He probably knows more about the common causes of acute illness than you do.

2. If you are only a locum preserve the *status quo*. Leave any 'improvements' to the permanent staff.

3. Don't write letters to committees without consulting your chief first. Your requests are then more likely to receive favourable consideration. Remember that a good unit ticks over on its human relations.

4. When another member of the staff has seen your patient previously be careful not to leave him uninformed or not consulted without reason. He and the patient may be pleased to meet again.

5. Never let the patient see that you are in a hurry.

6. Don't pooh pooh the patient's suggestions but give them courteous consideration.

8. Don't think it *infra dignitatem* to learn from Sister. She has had much experience.

9. Always see and speak to the patient reassuringly when he knows there has been a discussion of his illness even though you have to tell his relatives the sad truth. Kipling said, 'The most powerful drug in medicine is the spoken word.'

10. Tell the patient something and explain what you are going to do but whatever you say let it be in words he can understand. 'Except ye utter by the tongue words easy to be understood how shall it be known what is spoken. For ye shall speak into the air.' I Corinthians XIV, 9. The patient should never be left waiting, wondering and uninformed.

11. Use your unaided senses first. 'Eyes without the microscope, ears without the stethoscope, wits without the help of chemistry and radiology, not that we should deny ourselves the proper use of these, can often carry us a long way.' John Ryle. So order investigations with discrimination and use the least unpleasant ones first.

REGISTRATION

Registration procedures vary with the type of registration sought. You will have become provisionally registered before taking up your first post. Not every hospital authority in Britain asks about registration when making a contract to employ a doctor and this has led some to think that when they are given a contract registration has been taken care of. This is not so. The responsibility for becoming registered is yours and any employment before you are provisionally registered will not count towards full registration. Also you cannot be paid before you are registered.

In order to become fully registered you must first spend a year from the date of engagement (not qualification) in resident appointments (six months in medicine and six months in surgery, with a midwifery appointment counting as medical or surgical). At the end of each six months period you should obtain a certificate of satisfactory service from your chief and send the two certificates to the dean of the medical school which granted your medical degree or diploma. If they are accepted a Certificate of Experience will be issued with which you can apply to the General Medical Council for full registration. As the practice of all licensing bodies is not identical you should consult yours beforehand if there is any doubt about the acceptability of a post.

Doctors from overseas

Eligibility for provisional registration is determined by the qualification held, and for full registration by the qualification held and the experience gained. Hence a doctor must hold a recognised qualification and must have passed a test of knowledge of English before full or provisional registration is granted. Further information may be obtained from the General Medical Council.

Doctors holding overseas qualifications recognised for full and provisional registration and also other overseas qualifications, may apply for limited registration. This is granted for a specified period, either for one particular job or for a range of employment, but only in relation to appointments in which the doctor is supervised by another doctor who is fully registered. Limited registration may not normally be granted for a period or periods which amount in aggregate to more than 5 years. Before limited registration is granted for the first time a doctor must pass a test of knowledge of English and of professional knowledge and competence, the standard of which is related to suitability to hold a senior house officer post. Exemption from the test may be granted on a personal basis. The tests are conducted by the Professional and Linguistic Assessments Board. They occupy two days and comprise written and oral examinations but not at present a clinical test. They held at approximately monthly intervals in London, Edinburgh and Glasgow. A doctor is not normally admitted to the test unless he has completed a year's internship or equivalent service approved by the General Medical Council. You should consult the Council for advice on the types of employment which may be covered by limited registration. If an overseas doctor wishes to practise outside the NHS hospital service he must obtain a primary qualification recognised for full registration.

Registration fees are:

For doctors qualifying in the UK and other EEC countries: Provisional registration £20; full after provisional registration £30; full not after provisional registration £50.

For doctors holding qualifications granted overseas and recognised for full and provisional registration these fees are increased to £40, £30, and £70 respectively.

The initial fee for limited registration is either £25 or £50 depending on the circumstances. The renewal fee for an extension of limited registration is either £15 or £10 depending on the circumstances.

Doctors who qualify in the Irish Republic pay the same registration fees as those qualifying in the UK.

CASUALTY DUTIES

In some hospitals you may still be called on to do a period of casualty duty. Always notify the Receiving Room and the telephonist where you will be. Don't keep the patient waiting. If your hospital is equipped with the 'bleep' system don't forget to carry your receiver.

It is necessary to remind every houseman that in the case of a possible fracture, no matter how trivial the injury, he should always:

1. Have the patient X-rayed and see the wet film. Make sure that the part in question is on the film and having found a fracture look for a second one.

2. Give the patient appropriate treatment and refer him to the next fracture clinic.

3. See the radiologist's report later.

Never transfer a doubtful case after an accident.

When you give tetanus antitoxin you should advise the patient to return six weeks later for a course of three injections of tetanus vaccine (adsorbed) to give him lasting protection. You may give him a reminder card to facilitate this. Alternatively he should ask his doctor to give the injections.

MEDICAL RECORDS

The art of history taking is by far the most difficult part of the clinical examination to learn and great care should be spent on it. The patient's story should be elicited and written down legibly under the headings—History of the present condition; Past illnesses and Family history, though not necessarily in this order. In the case of an elderly person ask about his descendants as well as his forbears. His grandson's illness may provide the clue. Ask especially about recent residence and visits abroad. Take heed of a Medic-Alert bracelet or a personal details card or an entry, *e.g.* Allergy, on a passport. It is often best to receive the history *i.e.* to let the patient tell his story in his own way and in some cases alone in a quiet room. He may have to be coaxed to find words to express what he feels. You may then be able to make the 'second diagnosis', *i.e.* what it is that has really brought him to see you. Try to let him go at his own speed and do not let him feel that your time is more important than his. Be careful not to hinder or offend by your mode of address. Do not, for example, call your patient Grannie or Dad just because she or he is old. The lady who keeps the corner shop may like to be addressed in a familiar way but not so the vicar's wife. Try to size up the patient and sense which approach is best to make. A useful point to elicit early is what the patient has already been told. If when about to depart he says, 'By the way, doctor...' take due regard of what he then asks for it may be the whole clue to his troubles.

It is often helpful to learn whether the patient has relatives in the medical and nursing professions. Watch his face as he tells his story. Non-verbal communication never lies. Entitlement to a disability pension and its assessment may be relevant to the complaint. A photograph in the notes may be a great help later on. Failing this a brief 'pen picture' will help you to recall him. If you work in an unfamiliar part of the country it is useful to learn something of the common colloquial euphemisms. Try to make sure by cross examination that you and the patient have the same interpretation of common medical terms. The aphasic patient is not entirely beyond your reach. Some communication is possible with the help of pictorial cards issued by the Chest and Heart Association. In the case of a child find out from the parents before they leave whether he has had the various fevers and when, and also what immunizing injections have been given (this may have been done in the Receiving Room).

The various systems should be examined and the findings recorded In the case of a child let the parents see you examine him. It is well to write down your tentative diagnosis. Although in doing this it is a useful exercise to try to obey Occam's rule, 'It is vain to do with more what can be done with fewer'. the fact is that multiple diagnoses are usually necessary especially in the elderly. If your unit uses Problem Oriented (Weed) Medical Records you should learn from the Records Department the way to assemble the papers. It is well to initial or sign the notes. If you have to write a letter about the patient make it clear that you do so on behalf of your chief and send it promptly (*see p* 54).

As your notes may be subject to scrutiny by lawyers and other doctors you should avoid facetious comments, 'personal touches' and exclamation marks. Be careful what you write in any note you may give the patient to hand to his doctor. Patients sometimes steam open the envelope. With common surnames like Jones and Smith be very careful to record the correct forenames. If your hospital uses a unit system for records put the patient's unit number as well as his name on all his papers. You should also try to complete any items on the Details sheet which were omitted by the Admissions Officer, *e.g.* the National Health Service number.

A more elaborate examination should be made of the system or part which seems to be mainly involved. The usual sequence of Inspection,

Palpation, Percussion and Auscultation should allow time also for Contemplation. It is best to put 'right' and 'left' instead of R and L. The fingers should be described as thumb, index, middle, ring and little and the toes as hallux or big, second, third, fourth and fifth or little. As persons from some countries confuse toes and fingers it may be better to call them all digits. For almost every patient it is advisable to record the blood pressure, the result of urine testing and to have the chest X-rayed and the haemoglobin estimation made. These findings are often part of the 'data base' of POMR.

When certain diagnoses seem probable you may order the various investigations and perform the necessary manipulations on your own initiative, *e.g.* in septicaemia (blood culture), in possible syphilitic conditions (VDRL test*) and so on. But you should beware of ordering, without due forethought, a large number of tests or ones involving much labour in the laboratory on the off-chance that they may help. You should always explain to the patient what it is proposed to do. Acquiesence in the examination implies consent but for anything of an operative nature a form of consent should be signed (*see* *p* 32).

INCIDENCE AND PREVALENCE

It is well to have some idea about what is likely to be the incidence (number of cases arising) and prevalence (number of cases existing) of the conditions you hope to see in your hospital during the time you are an HP. You will probably encounter coronary thrombosis, congestive cardiac failure, cerebral vascular accidents, peptic ulceration, poisoning, bronchitis and rheumatoid disease. Other conditions bringing patients to hospital for investigation are obesity, thyrotoxicosis, chronic renal and liver failure and the problems of hypertension and loss of weight. In the children's ward you will see respiratory infections (presenting commonly as PUO), feeding problems, malabsorption and acute haemorrhagic nephritis (but rarely nephrosis). Rheumatic fever is hardly ever seen now. Your hospital's annual report, if any, will be worth perusal.

The incidence and prevalence figures for some conditions depend on the diagnostic criteria used. Diabetes is a good example. Six persons per 1000 of the population are known to be diabetics and there are probably about an equal number of persons with abnormal glucose tolerance. If post-prandial glycosuria (which occurs in 4 per cent of

*This (*p* 202) and also the TPHA (*p* 200) test is still referred to clinically as 'the WR' (Wassermann reaction) after the discoverer of the first serological test for syphilis (*see p* 286).

adults) is included the figure will be much higher. Disease incidence figures will also be affected by the age structure of the population. Where the proportion of elderly patients is high there will be a higher incidence of the disabilities of old age. Also some rare but non-fatal conditions diagnosed elsewhere will appear in later life in retirement areas and show as a high prevalence which is not due to any local cause. You should be clear whether any published incidence figures refer to a locality, England and Wales or the United Kingdom as a whole. The total number of some conditions in the whole country may be quite low but because of their interest and complexity they take up much space in textbooks though the chance of your meeting them will be small.

ABBREVIATIONS AND SLANG

Try to avoid abbreviations in your notes for another doctor may not understand them. FFP (full, free and painless) and RTA (road traffic accident) will be meaningful in the orthopaedic department and PMB (post-menopausal bleeding) in the gynaecology clinic but not elsewhere. ADL (activities of daily living) means nothing outside the rehabilitation department. It is in your patient's interest that your notes should be clear enough for anyone to read. Your own abbreviations may seem very sensible to you and you may think those of other people obscure and foolish but only very few abbreviations such as c.s.f. for cerebrospinal fluid and BP for blood pressure are universally acceptable. Some, though commonly used, are ambiguous such as CSU which may mean both a 'clean' and a catheter specimen of urine. Urine NAD is generally taken to mean that the urine was normal but the letters do not indicate what you tried to discover. It is better to say 'No albumin', 'No sugar' and so on. Private abbreviations such as SRI (seems rather ill) and GRS (godly, righteous and sober) are out of place in hospital notes. You will find help with difficult abbreviations in the *Dictionary of Abbreviations in Medicine and Related Sciences* by Edwin B. Steen (4th edn., 1978; price £2.50; Baillière, Tindall and Cassell) and *The Doctor's Shorthand* by Frank Cole (W. B. Saunders Co. 1970 price £5.00).

Slang and jargon should also be avoided. Their use is an untidy habit which easily develops in any profession. So also is the incorrect use of technical terms. Some of these have been wrongly used for so long that it seems hopeless to try to change. 'Doing a biopsy' for example is well understood though strictly removal of the tissue is distinct from looking at it. An i.v.p. is an excretion urogram and not an pyelogram but the abbreviation is here to stay. X-ray is a radiation of very short wavelength but is commonly used for the film. A convention is to write Xray for the rays and X-ray for the film. It is all right to use X-ray as a verb but when we want to refer to the record it makes, some call it a radiograph. At operation the surgeon does not 'remove the pathology' but the pathological tissue or organ. When nothing abnormal is found it is wrong to say that the pathology was normal.

EPONYMS

When you were in the dissecting room you were probably not encouraged to use eponyms for most anatomists preferred descriptive, if dull, terms. But in clinical medicine it is often convenient to use them (1) when, as in Menière's disease, the name does not commit you to any preconceived ideas of causation, (2) a scientific name would be long and cumbersome, (3) when, as in the cases of Horner and Argyll Robertson, the eponym has clearly come to stay, and (4) when, as in the case of Down's syndrome for mongolism, it is a more acceptable euphemism.

Eponyms give a historical flavour to your work and so you should try to know something about the men and women whose names they commemorate. But do not fall into the error of simply collecting eponyms and thinking that thereby your real knowledge is increased. Brief biographical details of names in this book are given on *p* 280 *et seq.*

PERSONAL RECORDS

Since, as a registered medical practitioner, you do not practise by the book or by authority but add to your knowledge of any condition by your experience of it you may like to have a follow-up plan to find out what happens to your patients. Personal records make this possible. How to keep them is for you to decide. It depends on how much time you can spare and how methodical you are. A simple note of the name, number and diagnosis will enable you to recall the record later. It is salutary to keep a 'black book' or private record of cases which went wrong and to peruse it quietly from time to time.

NOTES FOR DOCTORS FROM OVERSEAS

Britain. A geographical note

The sovereign state in which you are working is The United Kingdom of Great Britain and Northern Ireland, *i.e.* England, Wales, Scotland, the Isle of Man, the Channel Islands and six of the nine counties of

Ulster. Strictly, the term English does not include Wales and Scotland and the term British, though used officially as in British passports, is derived from the name of a Roman province long extinct. The people of Scotland call themselves Scots and their affairs Scottish but the English term Scotch for both is also correct. You may still see on some older documents the expression 'Wales and Monmouth' but for which purposes Monmouth was regarded as part of Wales became irrelevant when Monmouth was absorbed into the new county of Gwent.

'Doctor'

You may be puzzled because some of the medical staff are called Doctor and others Mister whereas in your own country all medical men and women are addressed as doctor. The title 'doctor' in Britain is generally taken to indicate that the holder belongs to the medical profession. He does not necessarily hold the degree of MD and is called Doctor more for the name of his profession than as a title of distinction. This usage is well founded in history. When most practitioners held doctors' degrees the title 'doctor' was extended to the few who did not to avoid any suspicion that they were not fully qualified. Consultants and senior registrars in surgery and gynaecology are generally called Mister—a curious survival of the days when surgeons were considered inferior to physicians. It is now the sign by which a surgeon can be distinguished from other medical men. In a few places house surgeons put on airs and call themselves Mister too!

BRITISH MEDICINE

If you qualified outside Britain you may at first feel bewildered by practice here. The British approach is essentially clinical and was well expressed by the late Sir James Spence of Newcastle when he said:

> The real work of a doctor is not health centres or public clinics or operating theatres or hospital beds. Techniques have their place in medicine but they are not medicine. The essential unit of medical practice is the occasion when, in the intimacy of the consulting room or sick room, a person who is ill, or believes himself to be ill, seeks the advice of a doctor whom he trusts. This is a consultation and all else in the practice of medicine derives from it.

You may learn something of the general aspects of medicine in Britain by reading articles and addresses. The following selection, some of which are classics, is offered.

Robert Hutchison (1928). The principles of diagnosis. *British Medical Journal,* i, 335.
Robert Hutchison (1938). Seven gifts. *The Lancet,* ii, 61.

Sir Henry Cohen (1943). The nature, methods and purpose of diagnosis. *The Skinner Lecture.* Cambridge University Press. (An abridged account appeared in *The Lancet,* 1943, i, 3.)

J. M. Lipscomb. (1949). On seeing the patient through. *The Lancet,* i, 171.

F. M. R. Walshe. (1950). On clinical medicine. (The Schorstein Lecture.) *The Lancet,* ii, 781.

G. P. Hardy-Roberts. (1951). Office manners. *The Lancet,* i, 1119.

Robert Platt. (1952). Wisdom is not enough. *The Lancet,* ii, 97.

J. W. Todd. (1952). Precision in diagnosis. *The Lancet,* ii, 1235.

Richard Asher talking Sense. Collected papers edited by Sir Francis Avery Jones (1974).

REASSURANCE

The importance of cultivating the art of reassurance justifies a few words on this topic. While reassurance involves your whole behaviour its main vehicle is your voice. This is more effective when its tone is right, for reassuring words lose value if uttered with an inflection of doubt. Beware of implanting doubt non-verbally as by frowning when you listen to the heart. While some claim that reassurance merely makes the doctor feel he has done something it should at least aim to leave the patient hopeful. If he knows he has obstruction to the blood vessels in his legs and asks what will happen keep your thoughts of gangrene to yourself and say you expect the blood will find a new way round. You will find opportunities for reassurance too in most clinical examinations. Try to anticipate the patient's fears. If you give him a wheel chair, for example, be sure to tell him that it does not mean that you think he will never walk again. You may appear to the patient to be constantly trying to find something wrong so it is well to say so when you find something right. Tell him his heart is fine while you keep quite about his knobbly liver. Sir John Parkinson (*p* 284) put this very well when he said that we doctors should take care to appear to the patient as counsel for the defence rather than for the prosecution. Strong reassurance is important therapy in conditions in which patients are aware of a sense of dying such as in vaso-vagal and panic attacks, adrenaline overdosage, labyrinthine vertigo, anaphylactic shock and some cases of angina.

Never tell a patient there is nothing more you can do for him but always let him feel on discharge that he may seek an appointment to see you again. A long-term follow-up appointment will make him feel he has not been abandoned. When put on medication for the rest of his life he can be given something to look forward to if he is told he will have to continue it till he is 86 especially if you let him feel he will live till then.

PATIENTS WHO DO NOT SPEAK ENGLISH

For simple instructions signs will suffice but to get a proper history the help of a colleague or nurse who speaks the language in question should be sought. The appropriate embassy or legation may help or The Institute of Linguists, 24A, Highbury Grove, London N5 2EA (tel. 01-359 7445) is pleased to supply the names of interpreters. The London Hospital (tel. 01-247 5454) can send interpreters in many languages to hospitals within reasonable distance. Many other hospitals keep registers of interpreters or 'language banks'. The British Red Cross Society's language cards may help (6 Grosvenor Crescent, London SW1X 7EQ, tel. 01-235 7131). As brief lists of phrases will not provide the details you want, the Polyglot Medical Questionaire by S. Chalmers Parry (2nd edn, 1972, Heinemann, £5.00) is recommended. It is in 27 languages and uses a digital system of communication.

SIGNS OF DEATH

In cases of long illness it is not difficult to decide that death has occurred, and as a rule it is the nursing staff who will inform you of it. Cooling, rigor mortis and post-mortem changes are the infallible signs but in most cases cessation of the heart beat is the most practicable sign. Death cannot be considered as certain until the heart has stopped beating for at least five minutes. Blood cells can be seen in clumps in the retinal vessels soon after death, the clear zones between them giving a 'cattle truck' appearance. As this may also be seen when the circulation is feeble or when the central retinal artery is blocked, it is not a completely reliable sign of death.

Test of death
If the relatives ask you to make a special test of death expose the radial artery at the wrist and cut it across. Having demonstrated the absence of bleeding apply a strip of plaster. Place the arm on the abdomen since if left at the side blood may seep out and cause an unsightly pool.

Brain death
The more difficult decision that the brain is dead though the heart beat continues will not be yours to make alone. It is rather that of those concerned in, but not in performing, renal transplantation. You should know, however, what evidence will be wanted to make a decision and help to assemble it. In a patient who is being kept 'alive' by a breathing machine the clinical diagnosis of brain death is based on a summation of many findings:

Complete apnoea and failure to re-establish breathing when the respirator is switched off for 3 minutes after previous ventilation with 100 per cent oxygen.

Widely dilated fixed pupils persisting for more than 24 hours except when the iris is bound down by adhesions or the patient is poisoned by mydriatic drugs.

No response to firm supraorbital pressure.

Absence of the normal 'doll's head' eye movements. (Normally ocular fixation is maintained despite movement of the head so that the eyes lag behind when the head is moved.)

No ocular movements after ice-cold water is syringed into one ear.

No corneal or gag reflex.

The ciliospinal reflex must be absent (dilation of the pupil on painful stimulation of the skin of the neck on the ipsilateral side). Even when present it may be hard to detect so look for it in a dim light using the plus 15 lens of the ophthalmoscope in order to detect the slightest movement.

These signs should be demonstrable at two examinations 12 hours apart. They should be interpreted with special care in a patient who is hypothermic or who has been poisoned by barbiturates.

The diagnosis of brain death may be supported by a completely flat e.e.g. record but even this is not infallible. Brain death produces a state of *'coma depassé'* (in which a patient has become a 'heart-beating corpse')—the best condition for removing the kidneys for transplantation if this can be legally achieved

HOW LONG DEAD?

It is wise when called to a patient whom you do not know and who has died suddenly and unexpectedly, to make observations on which an opinion may be given by you or someone else as to the time of death. (This is not necessarily the time of the injury which caused it.) The rectal or, failing this, the liver temperature (via a small incision under the right costal margin) should be taken. If the person has been dead for more than an hour or two a special low-reading thermometer may be needed. The rate of fall of body temperature after death is approximately 0.7°C per hour. Hence the number of hours since death is given by the formula:

$$\frac{36.8°C \text{ minus rectal (or liver) temperature}}{0.7}$$

Temperature readings should be taken hourly for a few hours.

The elderly and the young cool relatively quickly after death and the obese relatively slowly. So it is difficult to be exact and the result must be interpreted with caution. Some pathologists use a more elaborate calculation of the hour of death if provided with two temperature readings over a period of, say, 4 hours and the temperature of the surroundings.

Rigor mortis should be noted. A rough timetable is that is starts on the face in 6 hours and reaches the hands and feet at 12 hours; it stays 12 hours and takes 12 hours to pass off.

Post-mortem lividity due to movement of blood to dependent parts (hypostasis) begins within 1 or 2 hours of death and becomes fixed between 6 and 8 hours later.

DEATH IN THE AMBULANCE

You may have to see in the ambulance a patient, popularly known as BID ('Brought in dead') or DOA ('Dead on arrival'), to verify the fact of death. If you are uncertain see him in the casualty room. Consider the feelings of waiting patients in deciding how to act. Depending on where the patient lived you may accept the body in the hospital mortuary and tell the police or you may ask the driver to take it elsewhere when he will notify the police. Seeing a patient who breathes his last in the receiving room while you are trying to save him will not entitle you to certify the cause of death (*see pp* 14 and 15).

PERMISSION FOR NECROPSY

Under the Human Tissue Act 1961 permission for necropsy is vested in the hospital administration. But it is subject to objection from relatives to whom a dead body legally belongs and so it is good and usual practice to obtain permission (preferably written) from a close relative. Even if the deceased had given written instructions that a necropsy should be made the objection of a relative would prevent it. When no relative is 'reasonably' accessible the hospital authority (usually on the signature of a clinician or pathologist) can give permission.

In some hospitals a special person in the Records Department interviews the relatives but the job may fall to you. You may already have some idea of the attitude of the relatives and this may help you in the kind of approach to be made. If possible see the responsible relative in a quiet room and let him be seated. Allow him to discuss the illness and to ask questions. One of these will often give you the opportunity to say that a true answer can only be given after post-mortem examination. Failing this you should make a direct request for permission. Stress the fact that it is in the interest of the family and their descendants to know the exact cause of death. In most cases permission is readily given. (For necropsy on a Jew *see p* 30.)

If objections are raised do not make a begging approach or the relatives may feel they are doing you a favour in giving permission. Point out that post-mortem examinations are quite usual to confirm the cause of death; that the body will not be disfigured and that the face will not be touched (but *see p* 28.) Dispel any misconceptions that the body will be 'experimented on' or used for teaching anatomy (*see p* 28.) If you have some real doubt as to the cause of death you may say that you would find it difficult to sign a certificate and that one giving an 'uncertain' cause of death would be refused by the registrar and referred to the Coroner. It is unfair, however, to use the possible alternative of an inquest as a definite threat and the Coroner would resent his office being used for such a purpose. (Once a death has been reported to the Coroner a post-mortem examination can only be made on his order or with his consent. If you want to attend *see p* 20). When only a partial examination is allowed be careful to tell the pathologist lest he should do too much.

The relatives will probably ask to be told the findings. Take care not to forget such a request. See them or send them a letter written in simple non-technical language. Try to reassure them, if possible, that the cause of death was such that, in the present state of medical knowledge, no treatment could have prevented it. Remember that while the post-mortem shows what the patient died *with,* it does not always reveal precisely what he died *of.*

DEATH CERTIFICATES

It is usually your job to certify the cause of death on the prescribed form to the best of your knowledge and belief and without fee. (As it is the cause and not the fact of death that you certify the document is strictly a Medical Certificate of the Cause of Death.) Even if only provisionally registered you may certify in the hospital where you work but not elsewhere. Before signing your first death certificate you should study the *Notes and suggestions to certifying medical practitioners* in the front of the certificate book and the *List of indefinite and undesirable terms.* Precision in death certification is clearly desirable because statistics depend on it. If you are uncertain about any cause you should consult the *Manual of the International Statistical Classification of Diseases, Injuries and Causes of Death* (WHO, Geneva, 1970) which it is hoped is in the Records Office. Should you still be doubtful about the acceptability of a cause of death ask the Registrar of Deaths. (Some registrars have an office in the hospital.) To risk leaving him to refuse your certificate might cause inconvenience to mourning relatives and also would give them a poor opinion of your ability.

The issue of a death certificate is compulsory irrespective of whether the cause of death is natural or unnatural and, strictly, even though the death has been reported to the Coroner. The doctor who certifies must be the one who attended the deceased in his last illness. If he has gone away and there is no one else who could sign then the Coroner will have to be informed. 'Attendance' is not defined but is generally taken to mean seeing the patient on at least two occasions. The other requirements are that you must have seen the deceased within a reasonable period before death and the body after death. But if the period was 14 days or less you need not see the body after death and your certificate if otherwise in order will be accepted. (The period of 14 days is a Coroner's requirement.) Seeing the patient within 14 days of death and the body after death are alternatives except in the case of cremation certificates when both conditions must be fulfilled.

The section 'Seen/not seen after death by me' on the certificate is only included to help the Registrar to decide whether or not to report the death to the Coroner. If you see a patient moribund in the receiving room this will not entitle you to sign the death certificate. In such a case you should ring up the family doctor. He may be willing to certify but if he had not seen the deceased within 14 days and does not wish to come and view the body then the Coroner will have to be informed. In most hospitals it is usual when a death has been reported to the Coroner not to issue a death certificate. But the doctor has a statutory duty to certify and if the relatives desire it this must be done. The back of the certificate should be initialled at A (indicating that the death has been reported to the Coroner). In the rare instance of a Coroner deciding that there was no case for him to investigate, your certificate would be needed.

The procedure is as follows:

Observe the rules of your hospital about the time and place for signing certificates.

Fill in the cause of death and sign the certificate giving your *registered* qualification. Do not be unnecessarily verbose. Avoid imprecise terms and the word 'probably'. Be careful not to enter as the cause, albeit secondary, some condition such as an old and irrelevant fracture which would make the Registrar notify the Coroner, for this would only cause distress to the relatives. If bedsores are mentioned remember that an inquest will almost certainly follow. The conditions mentioned must be part of a causal chain. Put what the patient died *of* rather than what he died *with*. You could save trouble by including a note to say that a fracture which the relatives might mention to the Registrar was not the cause of death. Initial the back at A if the Coroner has been informed and at B if further information is offered later. When you are new to the hospital your signature will be unknown to the Registrar so it will help him if you also print it when you sign for the first time and every time if it is always hard to read. The Administrator will probably have notified the Registrar that you are about to take up a resident post. Do not forget to fill in the counterfoil.

The *Notice to Informant* lists the information which the Registrar will want and reminds the informant to give up the deceased's medical card. Although it is strictly the doctor's duty to deliver the certificate to the Registrar it is usually taken by a relative. Certification may await necropsy but if relatives want a certificate at once for funeral purposes it should be given and the back initialled at B. In cremation cases certification should only be made after necropsy.

Scotland now uses the same (international) form of death certificate as England and Wales in which the condition directly leading to death is stated first. The Scottish certificate also records deaths during pregnancy or within six weeks thereafter. In Wales certificates in the Welsh language can be used.

Deaths of war pensioners
When a deceased person has had a war pension it is in his widow's interest to state the cause of death if possible in such terms that it shows either a direct connection between the pensioned disability and the cause of death or that the disability could have materially hastened death. This may facilitate the widow's claim to the pension and obviate her need to appeal if she is not granted her husband's pension. A registrar is under no obligation to report a pensioner's death to the coroner and even if death was due to a pensioned disability this could have been a natural death, *e.g.* from tuberculosis. If a Coroner did decide that death was due to war service this might falsely raise the widow's hopes for the Secretary of State is not bound by a Coroner's verdict. So it is best in the case of a pensioner to issue a death certificate suitably worded but not, without other reason, to inform the Coroner.

The Coroner's certificate
Relatives may ask you whether reference to the Coroner will mean an inquest. Unless the death was clearly unnatural you can assume that there is a fair chance that an inquest will not be needed. If the Coroner decides that the doctor's certificate of cause of death is acceptable he

will issue pink form A which empowers the Registrar to register the death. This form is also used when the doctor who attended the patient is away and his locum has not seen the patient. Contrary to what is sometimes said the Coroner does not give permission to a doctor to sign a certificate of the cause of death. Alternatively the Coroner may order a post-mortem examination and if this shows that death was due to natural causes he will issue pink form B which authorises the Registrar to register the cause of death as shown by the post-mortem. The Coroner may also issue cremation form E which enables the medical referee of the crematorium to authorise cremation.

Cremation certificates
As the Registrar can only register a death if he has an acceptable certificate from a doctor or Coroner, permission to cremate will be refused by the crematorium referee if the cause of death is not definitely ascertained and usually by necropsy. Regulations about cremation have to be strict since it destroys all evidence. Of the seven necessary forms only three (B, C and F) have to be signed by doctors. Form B concerns the house physician and should be filled in with great care. It can now attract a fee. Question 5, 'Were you the ordinary medical attendant of the deceased?' should be answered NO. Question 6, 'Did you attend the deceased in his last illness?' must be answered YES. Your answer to question 7, 'When did you last see the deceased alive?' should indicate that you saw him not much more than 14 days before death and preferably less. Some doctors seem to think that when cremation is proposed the Coroner must be informed. This is not so. The method of disposal of a body is not the concern of the Coroner and all he does is to give evidence on form E which enables the referee to authorise cremation. The marginal note on form B of some crematoria that the Coroner must be told if the deceased was not attended within 14 days of death is not a statutory requirement and on the forms of other crematoria the interval is left to the medical referee. The answer to question 9 about the cause of death should repeat what was put on the death certificate but if necropsy has revealed some other cause this should be commented on at the foot of page 2 in such a way as to assist the referee. Form C which confirms form B must be signed by a practitioner of five years standing (excluding the year/s of provisional registration) who is independent of the doctor who signed form B. Strictly, the consultant in charge should decide who is to sign form C and he may do it himself. Objection might be made if forms B and C were signed by house physician and registrar as they are closely associated. (The need for form C has been questioned and there is no doubt that the examination which must precede it is often perfunc-

tory.) Form F authorising cremation is signed by the crematorium referee after scrutinising all the other forms.

Certification of deaths of babies

The crucial point is whether the baby had any separate existence. If it did then its birth and death must be registered however premature, *i.e.* even if born before the 28th week of pregnancy.

After the 28th week of pregnancy the birth of a child which does not show any sign of life after being completely expelled must be certified on a special Certificate of Still Birth by the doctor who was present at birth or who examined the body after death. Such a stillborn child may not be buried without a Registrar's certificate or a Coroner's order.

A child born before the 28th week of pregnancy which shows no sign of life has no existence at law and may be disposed of in any convenient way.

If you have any doubt as to whether the fetus may be required as evidence in any criminal investigation you should arrange for its preservation until the police have consented to its disposal.

NOTIFICATION OF THE CORONER

The Registrar of Deaths is the chief person whose statutory duty it is to report to the Coroner (or in Scotland the Procurator Fiscal) deaths which seem to him to come within the Coroner's jurisdiction. There is no similar statutory duty laid on a doctor as such though this duty may apply to him in this capacity as head of an institution. It may be that the Coroner has a social or moral claim on the doctor as on anyone else to report an unnatural death to him, but as such a claim would have no statutory basis and, as in any case the test of enforcement could not be applied, no claim of this sort is exercised. The doctor and, indeed, anyone else should be careful that he could not, by any intended act or omission, be held to be obstructing the Coroner in his duties. A system of cordial co-operation has grown up whereby 'Coroner's cases' are reported direct to the Coroner by the doctor and this is very convenient to all concerned. If you are in doubt as to whether the Coroner should be informed, consult your chief or the records officer or have a word with the Coroner's officer himself.

Deaths which it is the Registrar's statutory duty to report to the Coroner are:

1. Those where a registered medical practitioner was not in attendance.

2. Those where no certificate can be given.

3. Those where you did not see the deceased within 14 days before death or his body after death.

4. Those where the cause of death is unknown (*i.e.* where there is an 'uncertain' certificate).

5. Those where death was unnatural, unexpected, due to accident, violence or neglect or where it occurred under suspicious circumstances. Deaths attributable to or materially hastened by war *injuries* are included. (It is sometimes said that deaths from war pensionable *diseases* should be reported to the Coroner but this is not the case for although attracting pensions they may still be 'natural'.)

6. Those where death occurred after an operation.

7. Those where death was due to abortion, industrial disease or poisoning.
The current list of notifiable industrial diseases is long and includes dust diseases, various infections and poisonings. It should be consulted if need be.

8. Deaths of persons transferred from prison or police custody.

9. Stillbirths if no doctor or midwife was in attendance.

10. Deaths from any cause if the body is removed from the UK. (Burial at sea comes within the Coroner's jurisdiction. This is because the limit of the Registrar's district is low water level and not the three mile limit. Hence sea burial means removal from the ·UK. An exception is an area of sea less than 10 miles across which is regarded as British territory.)

Deaths of foster children have no longer to be reported but the possibility of the 'battered baby syndrome' must not be forgotten (*see p* 21).

Some Coroners ask that all deaths within 24 hours of admission to hospital should be notified to them, but this is a purely private local arrangement.

In a case of great clinical interest which, from some accident, comes under the Coroner's jurisdiction, the house physician should make a special request to be present at the autopsy. Otherwise valuable material, because of no medicolegal importance, may remain unexamined.

THE BRODRICK REPORT

The report of the Home Office Interdepartmental Committee on Death Certification and Coroners 1971 (The Brodrick Report) has been accepted in principle but the necessary legislation is still awaited. When it is made the information given above about death certificates and Coroners will be altered as follows. The doctor will be required to have seen the patient within 7 days before death and must view the body after death. If he cannot certify he must notify the Coroner, who will decide whether to hold an inquest or not. Only in cases of homicide, deaths of persons in custody and unidentified bodies will the Coroner be obliged to hold an inquest. The Coroner will be able to accept documentary evidence and so reduce the need for doctors to attend court. There will be no medical Coroners unless they are legally qualified also. Cremation certificates after death in hospital will be things of the past but outside hospital a second certificate from a member of a special panel will be needed. The certificate of the crematorium's medical referee will be abolished.

ATTENDANCE AT THE CORONER'S POST-MORTEM EXAMINATION

Although it is within the power and discretion of the Coroner to say who may be present and who may be excluded from a post-mortem examination there is usually no objection to your attending if you do so purely out of medical interest. If you had assisted at an operation or had given an anaesthetic to the deceased person and might be deemed to have been negligent you should not attend without the Coroner's consent. Under the Coroners (Amendment) Act 1926 you could send a representative.

THE HOUSE PHYSICIAN IN THE CORONER'S COURT

You will usually be told by telephone of an inquest but sometimes written notice is served. If you think allegations may be made against you or that you may be inculpated in some way it is well to be legally represented by your medical protection society. When several inquests are held on the same day and the evidence is not controversial a Coroner will sometimes take evidence from all the doctors early so that they can be released. A medical witness is generally treated with great consideration but he has no privilege of professional secrecy. If the time of an inquest is very inconvenient for you it is possible by a tactful approach to secure an alteration.

The rules of evidence which apply in other courts have to be relaxed in the Coroner's court. This is because much medical evidence which is accepted is technically hearsay only since it depends on reports of pathologists and other specialists. If cross examined you should answer Yes or No. If this is not possible you should explain in a way which shows that you are not being evasive or partisan. The Coroner should be addressed as Sir. Sometimes he sits with a jury. His decision or verdict on the person's death is concerned solely with the questions who is the person and 'when, where and by what means' did he meet his death. He is not concerned with liability but occasionally the jury may name someone as responsible for a death. More often the police have already started proceedings. Many a death is inquired into by the Coroner without an inquest if what you tell him shows that although unexpected it was natural.

THE HOUSE PHYSICIAN IN THE WITNESS BOX

You cannot escape having to appear in court if you have already seen and dealt with as a patient the person who is the subject of the hearing even though you did not think at the time that any legal action would ensue.

Notice to attend a court may take several forms. If there is any question of your being criticised in court you should certainly tell your medical defence society beforehand. The police may send you a note asking you to attend a magistrate's court voluntarily to give evidence for the prosecution. If necessary you can be summoned to attend and a warrant may even be issued in case of difficulty. In civil courts a notice to appear is sent by the solicitor preparing the case and as it cannot be refused with impunity it is called a subpoena (*i.e.* under penalty).

If you are involved in a High Court case it is a good plan to attend a hearing as a spectator beforehand so that you will not be completely strange to court procedure. A valuable book about this is Professor Keith Simpson's *Doctor's Guide to Court* (2nd edn, 1967).

When in the witness box try to answer all questions clearly and stick to the facts. Try not to be drawn out of the recognised field of your work and be calm and patient if attempts are made to discredit your evidence. Resist any temptation to take sides and leave advocacy to the advocates. You are there to help the court in its deliberations and not to achieve what you regard as a desirable end.

BATTERED BABIES AND OTHER INJURIES BY THIRD PARTIES

It is alas necessary for you to be alert to the possibility that trauma to a child may have been caused by his parents and you may meet such a case in Casualty. Your suspicions should be aroused when there has been delay between the accident and bringing the child to hospital; the parents are disturbed and their explanation inadequate or too plausible; there have been previous injuries or frequent attendances. Suspect any fracture under the age of 2 years (but remember that repeated 'natural' fractures can be due to the rare condition osteogenesis imperfecta). Be careful not by word or attitude to accuse the parents. The lines to take are:

1. Admit the child (with the mother if possible) for assessment and protection.

2. Tell the consultant paediatrician.

3. X-ray the part and preferably the whole skeleton but excluding the pelvis and spine unless specially indicated. There may be evidence of old fractures.

4. Test the blood for a bleeding disorder.

5. Obtain photographic evidence, black/white and colour. The photographer should make a signed statement of how he took the photo. The negative must be kept.

6. Tell the Social Worker.

If the parent refuses to leave the injured child in hospital the paediatrician may ask a Justice of the Peace to order the child's detention or inform the police or the National Society for the Prevention of Cruelty to Children. He may contact the Community Physician and the family doctor. The Local Authority may have an 'at risk' register in which cases or even minor and apparently 'normal' injuries are recorded. Reference to this may point to the diagnosis if there are previous or subsequent injuries. The family may be known to the welfare department on account of alcoholism or criminality.

The possibility also exists that elderly persons who fall down frequently have been assaulted by relatives ('granny battering') as well as that the true diagnosis is homicidal poisoning or injury.

MEDICAL REPORTS

If you are asked to write a report on a patient you should first get his written consent. You should write the report with anxious care and see that everything factual in it is correct. Do not, for example, say that you examined the patient 'today' when in fact you only spoke to his wife. If some facts would distress the patient then it is permissible to omit them from the copy which goes to him. A separate full report should be sent to the authority requesting it. Government departments have special rules about non-disclosure of information.

Although mainly for the consultant, you will find many useful notes on what points to record in the Notes in a small book *The Medical Report and Testimony* by Gerald H. Pearce, 1979.

MEDICAL CERTIFICATES

Medical certificates for National Insurance are, in effect, cheques drawn on public funds, and so you must be quite sure that what is certified is correct. A doctor's statement (Form Med 3) may have been issued by the family doctor but if not and the patient is in hospital it is your job to give it. You may sometimes issue a 'final' certificate. Whether a certificate is first, intermediate or final is determined by the way it is completed. When a patient is in hospital this is certified without a diagnosis on Form Med 10 (hospital in-patient certificate) by a doctor or authorised non-medical officer. It can be for 13 weeks in the first place. If a patient is fit for work on discharge Form Med 3 should be completed but if, as usually happens, he is referred back to his family doctor Form Med 10 should be used to show when in-patient treatment ceased. For a hospital out-patient the form used is the same as that of the family doctor (Form Med 3). It can only be signed by a doctor and a diagnosis must be given. It is for up to 28 days in the first place and after that for periods of up to 13 weeks (or longer in certain cases). Certification is in general the duty of the doctor who has clinical responsibility for the patient's treatment. The intricacies of certification are fully explained in document HM(71)40 issued in April 1971 and available in the administrator's office.

When you feel it inadvisable to disclose the nature of the disease you may give a vague diagnosis or simply write 'an illness' on Form Med 3. You should then complete the pink Form Med 6 (at the back of the certificate pad) to give the actual cause of incapacity in confidence to the Divisional Medical Officer. Failing this a vague certificate may result in the patient being referred to the Divisional Medical Officer though this is less likely to happen when the patient is in hospital than when he is at home. Some hospitals employ a clerk to make out certificates ready for your signature. The issuing of these certificates falls into category 1 (*see p* 26) and so no charge can be made for signing them.

If you think blank certificates (or prescription forms) have been stolen you should tell the hospital administrator. He may wish to change their form or colour for a time to render the stolen ones invalid.

Duplicate certificates for national insurance purposes may only be issued to replace lost certificates and they must be clearly marked 'Duplicate'. These rules do not apply to 'Private' certificates.

IF YOU ARE ILL YOURSELF

An old proverb says, 'He who treats himself has a fool for a patient', and so if you fall ill with something more than a common cold you would be wise to seek advice. There is often a consultant appointed to look after the hospital residents but you could, of course, consult anyone else. Even so, doctors often dose themselves with samples and deny themselves the standard of care they give to their patients. Although you are not legally debarred from prescribing drugs for your own use, if they are needed for your treatment it is best to get them through a colleague. You should not feel that any routine staff health checks and vaccinations do not apply to you. If you should persuade a radiographer to X-ray your chest (an unwise thing to do) and you show the film to your chief be sure to tell him it is yours. You may save yourself the nasty shock of hearing him think aloud about it.

Sick leave
A house physician absent from duty owing to illness is entitled to receive an allowance as follows: during first year of service, one month's full pay and (after completing four months service) two months half pay. During second year of service, two months full pay and two months half pay.

Sickness benefit
You should get a statement from your doctor on Form Med 3 (formerly called a medical certificate) and send it within 6 days (or 21 days if you have not claimed before) to the local office of the Department of Health and Social Security. They will decide your entitlement. Even though your pay goes on for a time when you are sick you should still claim sickness benefit lest you suffer certain immediate and delayed disadvantages. The personal flat rate of sickness benefit in 1979 is £15.75 per week.

Injury benefit
Many doctors and students do not know of their entitlement to compensation for injury at work. Examples of such injuries are: hand wounds when operating; bites on the fingers during manipulations such as gastroscopy; back strain from helping to lift a heavy patient; infections and their consequences and injuries from any accident whilst travelling on duty. If you think your incapacity results from any such injury sustained in Great Britain and Northern Ireland you should complete the relevant section on the back of the doctor's statement (Form Med 3) and send it with full details to the local office of the Department of Health and Social Security. You must also send an accident report to the hospital administrator. There are time limits for claims but it is best to assume it is never too late and to let the Insurance Officer decide. If your claim is accepted as an industrial accident, injury benefit of £18.50 per week (in 1979) will be paid until you are better or for six months, whichever is the shorter. After that

you may claim disablement benefit even though you are doing paid work again. Your loss of faculty will be expressed as a percentage by comparing you with a normal healthy person of your age but resulting loss of earnings cannot be taken into account. One hundred per cent disablement gives rise to a weekly payment in 1979 of £31.90.

Note on sickness and injury benefit abroad

If you seek experience in the United States or elsewhere abroad you should inquire about sickness and injury benefit when accepting the post and before you go. There is no federally sponsored national health care programme in the USA. Doctors there are generally expected to make private insurance arrangements though some hospitals offer these as fringe benefits. The ECFMG (p 49) has no part in these arrangements. Make sure that any health insurance is valid from the day of departure especially if by boat.

When you travel abroad as an ordinary citizen you may as an employed person obtain free treatment in some countries. (A general practitioner being self-employed would not be so eligible.)

HOUSE PHYSICIAN'S HAZARDS

It is well to know the special hazards of your work and to be aware of the common pitfalls which can lead to trouble.

Pitfalls

Here are a few reminders:

Missing a fracture, (p 4).

Head injury, cf. Drunk (pp 58 and 260).

The tourniquet. Having put it on don't expect someone else to take it off. Avoid using a transparent tourniquet.

Penicillin. Always ask about sensitivity.

Identification of the patient. Always be sure that the patient in question is the right one. Although mainly a surgeon's hazard a minor procedure carried out on the wrong patient may land you in trouble. A needle has been put into the chest unnecessarily because a chest film of another patient of the same name showed an effusion.

Giving information against the patient's interests, p 51.

Work beyond your responsibility,. p 34.

Illness or injury connected with your work, p 24.

Illness when working abroad, p 25.

Avoid being coughed upon. Some tuberculous patients with positive sputum are still around.

Don't let a patient's blood contaminate your skin. There is a risk of hepatitis. (*see p* 135).
Accidents in hospital, p 40.
Will you be sued for negligence?, p 34.
Use of apparatus. Be aware of how it may fail and think out beforehand what you would do if it did.

FEES

You may only receive fees for work which is outside the scope of the National Health Service, *i.e.* in category 2 of Appendix C of the *Terms and Conditions of Service* where details are set out fully. As most of your work falls into category 1, *i.e.* within the scope of the Service, you cannot expect to earn much from fees. Some fee-earning requests which may come to you are:

1. For medical reports on persons referred under the National Insurance (Industrial Injuries) Acts and by a medical board of the Department of Health and Social Security and other official boards.

2. For certain reports to the Coroner to help him decide whether to hold an inquest. A fee is only payable in areas where the local authority has made a schedule of charges.

3. For services as a witness. These fees vary according to the circumstances. If you are giving evidence for the Area Health Authority no fee is payable as you presumably attend court in your employer's time. Fees are payable when you are a witness in a legal action not involving the hospital. When a witness fee is not laid down by statute it is a matter for agreement and it is best to reach this beforehand.

4. For signing international certificates of vaccination.

5. For signing the 'first' certificate for cremation (Form B).

6. For notifying certain infectious diseases (*see p* 64) 25p.

ROUGH WEIGHTS OF CERTAIN ORGANS

(For ranges, sex differences and weights of other organs
see the table in the post-mortem room)

Thyroid	30g
Pancreas	90g
Kidneys	135g
Spleen	180g
Heart	300g
Liver	1.5 to 1.8 kg

DEATH BED WILLS

The house physician or anybody else (*e.g.* a nurse even if under 21) may witness the signature to a will. If asked, the house physician may help a patient to *make* his will if a solicitor is not available and if he is satisfied that the patient is of 'sound disposing mind'. If a special form is not used simply write *in ink* on plain paper as follows:

This is the last Will and Testament of Mr A. B., of...............in the county of...............I revoke all former Wills by me made. I appoint.......................to be the Executor(s) of this my Will.

(Here follow all bequests and instructions)

In witness thereof I have hereunto set my hand this...............day of...............one thousand nine hundred and.............Signed and acknowledged by the said A.B., the testator, as and for his (her) last Will in the presence of us, both present at the same time, who, at his (her) request, in his (her) presence, and in the presence of each other have hereunto subscribed our names as witnesses.
Testator's signature.
Witness's signature, address and occupation.
Witness's signature, address and occupation.

(Witnesses must not be executors or persons who benefit under the Will)

Dying depositions and declarations
You may be asked to take down the statement of a dying patient and though you are under no legal obligation to do so you would be wise to accede.

When the *patient* is in settled hopeless expectation of death the statement he makes is a **dying declaration.** It is limited to cases of homicide but is only admissible as evidence in reference to the person who makes it. What he says should be written down in full together with any questions used to elicit full information and their answers. The phrase, 'Having the fear of death before me and being without hope of recovery' must be included. The presence of a magistrate is unnecessary. The declaration should be signed by the dying patient if possible and by the person who writes it down. Witnesses are not necessary but are desirable.

When it is the *doctor* who thinks the patient is unlikely to recover but the patient is unaware of the imminence of death the statement taken is a **dying deposition.** A magistrate should be summoned and he will see that the legal requirements are complied with.

Eyes bequeathed for therapeutic purposes

If you learn that your dying patient has expressed a wish to donate his eyes you should obtain the consent of the relatives and friends and then inform the collection centre of the nearest hospital doing corneal grafting of the impending demise. If death has already occurred tell them as soon as possible. The hospital will, unless an inquest is likely, send out someone to collect the eyes. Pending removal instil drops of chloramphenicol 0.5 g/dl into each eye. Keep them closed lest the cornea dries. Have the body kept in the refrigerator.

Body bequeathed for dissection

If you find that a dying patient has expressed a wish that his body should be used for dissection you may wonder what should be done. The relatives or the doctor should telephone HM Inspector of Anatomy, 16–19 Gresse Street, London W1P 1PB (01-636 6811 ext 3572 or 3576, or after office hours Duty Officer, DHSS Headquarters, 01-407 5522 ext 7407). In Scotland telephone Anatomy Office, Division IIIB/B2, Room 235, St Andrew's House, Edinburgh EH1 3DE (031-556 8501 ext 2936) or the nearest medical school. In Wales or Northern Ireland contact the Professor of Anatomy. Full instructions will be given. An ordinary death certificate is necessary. The doctor supplying it will be questioned and a decision whether to accept or not will be made at once. If accepted the green Disposal Certificate, issued when any death certificate is accepted by the Registrar, is given to the undertaker sent by HMIA. Forms AA1 and AA4 will be sent for completion by the doctor. There is no fee and no donation to any person or charity is necessary. Acceptance cannot be guaranteed for it depends on the current needs of the medical school and the many factors such as a diffuse disease or a post-mortem examination which may make the body unsuitable. Once accepted, however, disposal of a body would not be at the relatives' expense.

Donated (cadaver) kidneys

You may wonder what to do if you find your very ill and possibly moribund patient carries a signed kidney donor's card. First consider acceptability. Kidneys may be medically acceptable if the donor is between the ages of 2 and 65 and is not suffering from cancer outside the c.n.s., diabetes, collagen diseases, established renal infection or severe septicaemia. Kidneys are probably unsuitable if there has been hypotension for more than 12 hours leading to oliguria or if the patient has been on a noradrenaline drip. (In practice most donors have suffered a head injury or a subarachnoid haemorrhage.) Admit the patient to the ward or intensive care unit and keep his breathing going by intermittent positive pressure ventilation. Phone the National Organ Matching Service in Bristol (0272 62821) or the nearest Transplant Team for instructions about what blood to send where for tissue typing. You may be asked to give heparin 5000 units, frusemide 250 mg and mannitol 100 g to resuscitate the kidneys. What follows will be in the hands of the team. Even if the recipient's hospital is nearby never contemplate transfer of the donor to it.

You should be aware of the legal position re permission to proceed. The Human Tissue Act 1961 enables the person lawfully in possession of the body, such as someone in a post designated by the Area Health Authority, to allow the kidneys to be removed. Actual possession of a body is not the same as the right to possession of it. If a person with this right appears the Area Health Authority cannot dispose of the body. It can only do so if, having made such reasonable inquiry as may be practicable, no surviving relative objects. When the deceased (to express his wishes) and the next of kin (to indicate their consent) have signed a kidney donation card this is sufficient. The transplant team may relieve the HP of the delicate task of asking the relatives. If a potential donor's condition is deteriorating rapidly you would be wise to identify the relatives quickly and ask the police to bring them to hospital.

ON CERTAIN RELIGIOUS MATTERS

The house physician is not specially concerned with the religious aspect of the lives of his patients when in hospital. Indeed he is usually unaware of their religious beliefs and these as recorded on the details sheet are not necessarily accurate or more than nominal. The house physician should be on friendly terms with all visiting clergymen and religious workers and help them in every way possible in their work. Only urgent and essential treatment should delay their access to patients.

Church of England patients
The clergyman is usually informed by the relatives that the patient is in hospital or by the ward sister at the patient's request. When Holy Communion is administered a table or locker with a white cloth and a medicine glass of water are provided at the bedside behind screens. When anointing is requested a little cotton wool should be put out also.

Roman Catholic patients
The priest is usually summoned by the nursing staff but it is well that the house physician should know how and when this is done. The

priest should be informed as soon as a Roman Catholic patient is placed on the Seriously Ill List. It is helpful if he can be told if the patient is unconscious. If a Roman Catholic patient is brought in dead or quickly dies the priest should be informed nevertheless. Extreme Unction or Last Rites are administered to seriously ill patients and for this it is usual for the ward sister to provide the same materials as for Church of England patients. A small vase of flowers may be included. Similar preparations are made for Holy Communion. Fasting is no longer a requirement and medicines need not be omitted.

Jewish patients
When a Jewish patient dies the body should not be removed to another room but should be kept in the ward at least until dawn and preferably not taken to the mortuary until a watcher arrives. In the case of a moribund Jewish infant no special measures are called for and after death the procedure is as for an adult. Post-mortem examinations are usually only performed on Jewish patients on the Coroner's order.

Moslems
During the Islamic fast of Rosa in the 30 day month of Ramadan smoking and the taking of all food, drink and medicines are proscribed between dawn and sunset. The dates and length of fasts vary since Ramadan is calculated on a lunar cycle. Medical treatment would exempt a Moslem and allow substitution of fasting days later but if your patient did not wish to do this you could prescribe drugs which could be taken in single or twice daily doses before dawn or after sunset.

Patients of other denominations
The Minister concerned will make his requirements known to the ward sister.

BAPTISM

The house physician should know what to do if faced with a request to baptise a very ill child. The clergyman should be summoned if possible and baptism by a lay person, such as a doctor or a nurse, should be performed only in a case of necessity. The reality of the necessity, however, is for the person performing the baptism to decide.

Baptism may be administered by any sane person, male or female, whether he or she has been baptised or not and irrespective of religious belief provided it is intended to do what the Church does. Two things are necessary: (1) invocation of the Holy Trinity, and (2) the use of water. If these are used baptism is valid. Godparents are unnecessary in an emergency.

The doctor's fingers moistened with water should touch the child's forehead while he says 'I baptise thee (A) in the name of the Father and of the Son and of the Holy Ghost' (Roman Catholics require the water to be poured). A name is not necessary for emergency baptism.

If there is any doubt particularly in the mother's mind as to whether baptism has already been performed or whether the child is alive, the baptism should be made conditional by prefacing the above words with 'If you can be baptised....' The clergyman of the parents' denomination should be informed afterwards.

MEDICO-LEGAL NOTES

Many doctors are very vague about certain medico-legal points and so a few selected subjects of general interest are briefly mentioned here. When any circumstances may, even remotely, involve the doctor in medico-legal difficulties the best advice he can be given is that he should inform his medical defence society at once of all the circumstances in detail. He must not have neglected, of course, to pay his annual subscription and every newly qualified doctor is strongly advised to do this by Direct Debit. (A pre-registration house physician can join a medical defence society on taking up his appointment and is entitled to full benefits and privileges.)

OWNERSHIP OF CLINICAL RECORDS

Clinical notes and X-ray films are strictly the property of the Area Health Authority. When a solicitor or other third party asks to see them for some legal reason not involving the hospital the appropriate consultant's permission is sought and the notes are usually sent. A request to see them for no clear reason would probably be refused. Committee members may not peruse notes just to satisfy personal curiosity.

Occasionally a patient prefers that certain facts should not be recorded in the notes. Then and also when you feel it would be prudent to omit them, either nothing should be written down in the notes or the papers should be kept in a private file to which you alone have access.

A private patient's X-ray films are generally regarded as the radiologist's property though he often sends them with his report at the request of the patient or his doctor.

CONSENT FORMS

Normally on the legal principle *Volenti non fit injuria* consent is
implied for any treatment which the patient willingly accepts. In most
cases consent is a mere formality and implicit in the behaviour of the
patient. Whether consent is written, verbal or implied will vary with
the circumstances but in all serious situations written consent is
necessary. Without consent treatment constitutes an assault in law and
so when an operation seems likely it is well to have a consent form
signed in good time. This is generally arranged by the ward sister but
you should verify that it has been done. The person giving consent
must understand what he is consenting to and so appropriate explana-
tions must be given (*see p* 2, *para* 10). To obtain consent for cardiac
catheterisation, for example, by saying it was just a needle in the arm
would be 'consent by trickery' and invalid. The use of 'blanket'
consent forms is no longer acceptable. It is not legal for a parent to
consent to any investigation of his child which is not to the child's
benefit, *e.g.* removal of normal tissue for biopsy for research purposes.
In gynaecological conditions consent sometimes raises difficult problems beyond the realm of the house physician. The only exception to
expressed consent is an emergency endangering life, for then the law
presumes the patient's consent on the theory that in such circumstances he would consent if able to an operation in his best interests. In
English law there is no rigid rule which makes a minor incapable of
giving his consent. The consent of the parent or guardian should
normally be obtained before operation on a minor under 16 but the life
of the young patient should not be jeopardised by waiting for formal
consent if the need for operation is urgent. It would be wise, however,
to obtain first confirmation of your opinion from several doctors.

RESPONSIBILITY OF HOUSE PHYSICIANS

There are certain duties which you can properly perform without
reference to your chief, *e.g.* lumbar puncture in possible meningitis.
There are other duties about which your chief should first be consulted. When you engage in a procedure which is well within your
competence and skill and which is within the general delegation which
you enjoy then you can be held responsible for all that flows from that
procedure. So long as you restrict your activities to the orbit within
which it is usual for a house physician to act then your chief can
repudiate responsibility for any mishap. As he cannot do all the work
himself you are there to help him but he has a responsibility for the
supervision of your work and so might be involved also in any action
against yourself.

Under the provisions of the Medical Act 1956, sub-section 17, a pre-registration house physician is entitled only to carry out duties assigned to his appointment, *i.e.* he can only practise in hospital.

It is not usually your responsibility to treat members of the nursing staff. If they ask you to prescribe for them or to order investigations you should refer them to the doctor who looks after resident nurses. Non-resident nurses should be told to consult their own doctors.

MINIMUM TIME OFF-DUTY

The Terms and Conditions of Service January 1971 as subsequently altered allow time off duty for senior registrars and lower grades as follows: two nights out of three (normally Monday to Thursday); two week ends out of three, (being the nights of Friday, Saturday and Sunday and the days of Saturday and Sunday). You will work to a 40 hour week contract with extra payment for 'overtime'.

In any hospital there must be considerable flexibility of duty rotas to allow off-duty time. All questions of off-duty and leave are dependent on the exigencies of the service and many doctors find they cannot always get time off because of some seriously ill patient. You are advised to take a reasonable and professional view of this and not to enter into acrimonious disputes about it. Human nature is such that foolish behaviour will be remembered while your good qualities are easily forgotten. It sometimes pays to be a willing horse. As you do not yourself negotiate the terms of your contract this is a one-sided 'take it or leave it' arrangement. You will be wise only to seek alterations in it through the proper negotiating channels while you get on with the job and gain all the experience you can.

Annual leave
An HP gets four weeks leave in a year and an SHO and registrar five weeks, plus national holidays or days in lieu. The year runs from the date of your appointment. Leave cannot be carried forward. You cannot take extra pay in lieu of leave and you cannot be your own locum. You would be ill advised to try to work in your own hospital during leave. But if you worked when away from hospital, *e.g.* in a practice or on a ship, nothing would be said. In some posts you will be required to cover the annual and study leave of a colleague. Such extra work is remunerable.

Study leave
A post-registration HP and an SHO may take day release with pay and expenses for the equivalent of one week during university terms or

with pay and expenses for up to a maximum of 30 days a year (from the date of appointment). Leave to sit examinations is allowed at the discretion of the Regional Health Authority. A pre-registration HP is allowed reasonable time off within working hours to attend conferences and rounds within the hospital. If you are uncertain of your entitlement ask the hospital administrator.

LOCUM WORK WHEN OFF-DUTY

It is not advisable for you to seek locum work when on leave or off-duty for you could not knowingly be so employed by a Area Health Authority and in any case payment could be withheld. You may be asked to take an evening surgery to help out a single-handed doctor in need but, although limited permission has been granted for this 'moonlighting', it would only be feasible occasionally and not on a regular basis. Your first obligation is to your chief and the duties of your post and, while theoretically the consent of the Area Health Authority would be necessary, no action would be likely to ensue over an isolated instance unless the work of the hospital suffered. Only a fully registered and not a temporarily or provisionally registered doctor or one in a pre-registration post could undertake such work. You could work outside the NHS when on annual leave as, for example, as a doctor on a pleasure cruise or in a country of the European Economic Community with impunity and both would provide new experience and enjoyment. But you should not lose sight of the fact that leave is primarily for rest and recreation.

SUED?

What is the risk of your being sued for negligence? In law negligence is judged by the standard of competence of an ordinary reasonable man. If you undertook some procedure which required specialist knowledge and skill outside your field you would be negligent if you bungled it even though you did your best. But provided you acted with reasonable care and skill appropriate in the particular circumstances you would not be found guilty of negligence. This means that you must follow the normally accepted practice of your profession at the time and, of course, it is your duty to keep reasonably abreast of modern practice. You are not infallible and if you make a mistake you will not be negligent provided you brought reasonable skill and care to bear upon the matter in hand.

Sometimes a patient, by his own negligence, may contribute to his injury. This is particularly so in accident cases and it is helpful to keep a careful note of the sequence of events in such cases as this may assist in reducing the size of the patient's claim. If a patient refuses to follow your instructions after an accident you should, after carefully explaining the position, withdraw from the case. In this way you establish contributory negligence and make any liability apportionable between you and the patient.

HOUSE PHYSICIANS WHO ARE MARRIED WOMEN

As confusion may arise, *e.g.* on certain certificates, if a registered medical practitioner does not use the name by which he or she is registered with the General Medical Council, a married woman practitioner should continue to use her maiden or other name in which she was originally registered. She can change her name in the Medical Register by sending her written request with her marriage certificate to the General Medical Council, 44 Hallam Street, London, W1N 6AE. No fee is charged.

STUDENTS

In many general hospitals whose staffs are prepared to accept responsibility for their supervision final year students now work, with the consent of their deans, for periods of up to about four weeks, usually in the vacations. The legal position of the student has been little tested but on general principles he would be liable for his own negligence. As he acts with the consent, even tacit, of the Hospital Authority, this body would be vicariously liable. The consultant for whom the student acts might be liable too if he neglected to supervise. Although he sometimes acts for a registered house physician he is never a 'locum' for an absent HP and responsibility in the absence of a qualified locum devolves on another member of the medical staff. A student cannot sign death certificates or prescribe, though he may administer, controlled drugs. He must not work unsupervised in a casualty department and should always be instructed and encouraged to seek help when in doubt. If he attempts something beyond his competence he does so at his peril. He cannot look for protection to a medical defence society and his service (and incidentally that of a qualified locum) cannot be reckoned for purposes of seniority. A student assisting voluntarily at the request of the Hospital Authority receives free lodging but must pay for his meals. He must pay contributions for insurance to the Hospital Authority on his honorarium (at the time of writing, 50 per cent of the minimum scale for house officers) but not on his residential emoluments. He would be entitled to claim sickness and injury benefit (p 24).

It is well to take heed of what a student finds out. A patient may confide in him something which he would not tell you or Sister perhaps because he feels that no threat of decision making is imposed.

CLINICAL ATTACHMENT FOR OVERSEAS DOCTORS

Overseas doctors wishing to practice in NHS hospitals must success-fully complete an attachment (normally four weeks) or obtain exemp-tion from it. Doctors should apply to the Central Clearing House, Department of Health and Social Security, Eileen House, 80–94 Newington Causeway, London SE1 6EF (01-703 6380 ext. 3827). Attachment arrangements will not be completed until the Clearing House is aware of their registration position. Doctors seeking limited registration will have their attachments arranged once it is known that they have been succesful in the PLAB test (Professional and Linguis-tic Assessments Board) or have been exempted from it. Doctors applying for full registration will have their attachments arranged following success in the language component of the test. Attachment is not offered until doctors have obtained full registration.

Attached doctors are paid at half the rate of pay of a house officer on first appointment. Accommodation is free but meals have to be paid for.

Doctors eligible for provisional registration only should obtain the experience necessary for full registration before coming to Britain as attachments are not normally offered until a doctor is fully registered.

MEASURES UNDERTAKEN BY THE NURSING STAFF

The house physician should remember that if he asks a nurse to carry out some procedure, e.g. taking of blood or giving an i.v. injection which is outside the scope of her normal duties he takes the responsi-bility. He should only do this if he has satisfied himself by personal observation of the nurse's competence. If he is doubtful about this he should use the needle himself. Some hospitals keep lists of nurses and technicians who are permitted to use i.v. needles. Nurses who hold the ophthalmic certificate are qualified to remove corneal foreign bodies.

PATIENTS WHO REFUSE TREATMENT

If after explanation a patient refuses to stay in hospital or to have treatment as advised the fact should be recorded in the notes. Before he leaves he should be asked to sign a statement that he is taking his own discharge against medical advice. If he cannot write he may make an X witnessed by your signature and this 'signing by witnessed mark' is legally valid. You cannot compel him to sign. If he refuses you should record this fact also in the notes. The refusal to allow an emergency operation on a patient under 16 could be over-ruled by the doctor if life was in the balance. If you feel that the patient is mentally ill and particularly if he has made a suicidal attempt you should seek the psychiatrist's opinion.

Jehovah's Witnesses
Very occasionally you may meet a member of this sect who refuses blood transfusion on religious grounds. Even if you regard his reasons (Genesis 9, v. 3, 4) as hair-splitting nonsense you should not approach the problem in an intolerant way. Talk to the patient in the presence of a witness and warn him of the dangers. If he cannot be persuaded to change his mind ask him to sign a witnessed statement of refusal. It is for your chief to decide on further treatment. The patient must not be transfused without his consent for no one is obliged to preserve his life by special or extraordinary measures. If a patient lays down a condition of no transfusion your chief may prefer to refuse the case but whether avoiding the responsibility in this way is justified is a moral issue for him to decide. We all have a duty to do all we can to preserve a patient's life and health and it may be preferable to get round the problem by regarding it as one in which ideal treatment is impracticable and to use a plasma expander instead of blood. You should make full records and include a note as to whether the patient was in full possession of his faculties.

In the case of a baby with haemolytic disease of the newborn the procedure of bringing a magistrate to the bedside in order to transfer custody of the child to the Children's Officer who would then grant permission for transfusion is a strategem to be discouraged. It is not approved by the DHSS and its legality would be doubtful for the order could not be subject to appeal as other legal decisions are. You would not stand by and let a baby die for want of transfusion and if you acted in good faith, albeit without legal sanction, the defence societies have guaranteed to support you in any action for assault. Even if this were sustained the damages would probably be minimal particularly if the child's life had been saved.

PATIENTS AND TEACHING

Formal teaching of both undergraduates and post-graduates takes place nowadays in many hospitals and many patients are also used as subjects in professional examinations. Most patients know this and accept it. Their treatment is in no way conditional on their agreement to be subjects for teaching, however, and you must never attempt to make it so. You must respect any patient's unwillingness to be used for teaching. He must be treated as a person and not impersonally as an object. It is wise when you arrange a teaching session or demonstration to let it be apparent that he is a willing collaborator (*see p* 2 *para* 10).

THE SUICIDAL PATIENT

It is sad and embarrassing to remember too late that your patient showed signs of suggesting that he was saving up an overdose or going to throw himself out of the window. You should therefore learn to spot the potential suicide and take preventative action. Most suicides indicate their feelings to someone so always take serious note of any self deprecating thoughts and expressions of suicidal intent particularly in the older adult. Factors which indicate a serious risk are: (1) family history of suicide, (2) history of previous attempts, (3) depression with self reproach, (4) isolation and loneliness, (5) severe physical illness.

Pending psychiatric help take commonsense precautions such as removal to the ground floor and giving drugs in liquid form or as opened capsules and in single doses. Lastly, never let a patient who is even a slight suicidal risk leave hospital without a psychiatrist's opinion. Even if your suspicions are unfounded it is better to make a mistake which allows for safety than have your patient commit suicide. Remember too that the unsuccessful suicide may bring an action against the hospital for not preventing him from damaging himself.

The failed suicide

Attempted suicide ceased to be an indictable offence in 1961 and so you are under no legal obligation to report it to the police. If you find a note in the patient's pocket you should regard its contents as confidential and keep them to yourself. You do not have to hand any tablets found to the police or anyone else but you may wish to send them for identification. If there is a police investigation, as in the case of a 'suicide pact', you should seek advice on how to proceed from your defence society.

ADMISSION TO A PSYCHIATRIC HOSPITAL

You should be aware of the general procedure under the Mental Health Act 1959 and how you may be concerned in it.

Informal admission

This is the preferred method for it preserves the freedom of the patient, who is sent to hospital in the ordinary way. The doctor must be satisfied that he is not unwilling to go. If age 16 or over his wishes override those of his parents or guardians. Occasionally an informal patient decides to leave the psychiatric hospital before the Local Authority Social Worker (LASW) arrives. If it is thought he may be a danger to himself or to others a recommendation on Form 6* by a consultant will allow detention for 72 hours. As there is now no essential difference between a general and a psychiatric hospital as far as admission is concerned detention in a general hospital, if thought necessary, can be achieved for 72 hours under section 30. The forms should be sent to the hospital administrator.

Compulsory admission

Admission for prolonged treatment requires two forms to be completed—one by an approved doctor.

Emergency admission under section 29 is used when a psychiatrist's opinion cannot be awaited. The LASW for the area where the patient is should be called. He will get in touch with the relatives and provide the necessary forms. He or a relative signs Form 2 (the application for admission). A doctor who knows the patient signs the medical recommendation but you could sign this yourself in an emergency. The patient can be detained for 72 hours. He cannot be discharged by a relative and usually a second recommendation is made during the 72 hours for admission for observation under section 25.

The procedure under the Mental Health (Scotland) Act 1960 is basically the same as but differs in detail from that in England and Wales. Transport is arranged by the Scottish Hospital Service and not by the LASW. Compulsory admission involves approval by the sheriff.

Informing the police. When a patient has been brought to a psychiatric hospital by the police or is reported by them to have been violent and cannot be detained or is taking his discharge then it is now a requirement that these facts must be reported to the police and the LASW.

The **disturbed patient in the Casualty Department** who refuses to accept treatment and leaves hospital presents an urgent problem. The simplest procedure is to ask the police to use their powers under Section 136 of the Act to remove the patient from a public place to a place of safety, *e.g.* a hospital, for examination. He can

*From Shaw & Sons Ltd, Shaway House, Lower Sydenham, London SE26 5AE (01-722 5131).

then be dealt with as already outlined. Alternatively the police may themselves call the LASW to see the patient outside the hospital, *e.g.* the police station.

Note. Completion of the forms does not mean that admission will necessarily follow. The Area Health Authority through its senior staff always retains the right to control admissions. You should therefore find out the admission procedure at your local psychiatric hospital.

COMPULSORY ADMISSION TO A GENERAL HOSPITAL

You may occasionally have a patient whose compulsory admission has been effected under section 47 of the National Assistance Act 1948. To achieve this two doctors (a general practitioner and a consultant employed by the Local Authority) must certify to a Justice of the Peace that the person (1) is suffering from grave chronic disease, (2) is in need of care and attention which he cannot provide himself or receive from anyone else, and (3) is living in insanitary conditions. Detention in hospital is for a period of up to 21 days.

ACCIDENTS IN HOSPITAL

Should an accident befall any patient, visitor or member of the staff go promptly when summoned. Enquire into the circumstances, examine the patient fully and order any necessary X-ray examination. Make a full, frank and factual report at the time preferably on a special form and send it to the hospital administrator. Include a note of the place where the accident occurred. In slipping cases it is often helpful to note the condition of the floor and shoes. You should treat the report as a confidential statement for the use of the solicitor of the governing body in case any claim is made. Do not make a copy as this would prevent its being treated as a privileged document. Bear in mind, however, that such a report may be admissible in evidence in subsequent legal proceedings and endeavour to make it as accurate and complete as possible. You should, of course, take all steps to reverse the consequences of the accident. If it seems that you may be involved as a cause inform your medical defence society.

WHO IS YOUR 'BOSS'?

If you are from overseas you may wonder who of the many lay and medical people around you in hospital is your 'boss', *i.e.* for whom are you working and to whom are you responsible. The days have gone when everything that happened in some hospitals was, in theory, the responsibility of one man—the Medical Director or Superintendent. There is now no such a medical executive and in general the hospital is run by a concensus group, the District Management Team of the Health District, which reaches its decisions by agreement after discussion and persuasion. Each person is responsible for what goes on and his own sphere. House physicians and registrars are employed and paid by the Area Health Authority to whom they are responsible except in clinical matters. (In the case of consultants and senior registrars it is the Regional Health Authority.) All doctors are subject to the current terms and Conditions of Service. Clinical direction is only given to you by your senior medical colleagues (registrar, senior registrar and consultant) and in this sense for your professional work the consultant is your 'boss'.

WARD PROCEDURE

After the nursing staff the house physician is the person who has more contact with the patient than anyone else. He becomes, so to speak, the 'family doctor' for the patient while in hospital. Everything that happens to the patient goes through him and so he acts as a liaison between various departments. You must not assume that you only have to deal with bedside matters. Your job is to see that all necessary investigations are made and that the patient understands what is happening and is satisfied. You are responsible for the patient as a person and not as a vehicle of some disease process. So do not be adverse to doing odd jobs for him (or for Sister). Always listen with respect to the suggestions of relatives for only too often their apparently unreasonable ideas turn out right. If there are relatives in the medical or nursing professions you may need to exercise great tact. When you talk to the patient stand at the bedside and not at the end of the bed and let it appear, even though you are in a hurry, that you have plenty of time to listen. So don't look at your wrist watch in front of the patient. Beware of inappropriate conversation at the bedside of the supposedly comatose patient (*see* p 260).

THE HOUSE PHYSICIAN'S ROUND

You will probably be the first doctor to see the patient after admission. He may think you are the doctor whose name is printed on the card over his bed. So disillusion him early rather than disappoint him later. In many hospitals doctors wear name badges. A booklet may be provided telling the patient about the hospital and the patient may want to ask you questions about it. Be patient with him for what appears commonplace to you may be strange and worrying to him.

It is the usual procedure for you to make a round of all your patients every day and also a night round. See every patient however briefly so that none feels he is forgotten or neglected. It is a good plan not to go round in the same direction each time so that the last patient you see, when you are perhaps hurrying, is not always the same one.

You are the doctor who has most to do with the patient and the one who plays a major part in giving the hospital its reputation. So cultivate a cheerful and reassuring manner and remember what Osler said about the patient who got better—'Doses of optimism lavishly prescribed by the house physician cured him'. It is very important that each patient should feel satisfied with his treatment and the explanation given to him. If he is not satisfied his treatment, however good technically, is incomplete. The days when the patient was kept in the dark have gone. Today's patient should be told what is happening in words he can understand. Many do not know how to ask the right questions and so do not complain. Others complain too much and it is wise to develop the facility of detecting them early and of taking steps to avoid trouble—often by seeking a second opinion.

THE CHIEF'S ROUND

In most hospitals a full ward round by all members of the unit takes place at regular intervals. See that everything—reports and X-ray films—is ready for it. You should be *au fait* with all details of the illness. When you have seen a laboratory report it is a good idea to initial it or otherwise show that you have taken some action on it. The occasion of the chief's round is a good one for you to change your white coat.

The ward round must be an orderly affair. Your chief may not have seen the patient before so do not show restlessness as he goes over the history which you already know or show how bored you are by looking out of the window. You may be itching to look at the X-ray film or the e.c.g. record but you should be watching and learning while your chief is examining the patient.

Try to avoid argument about diagnosis and treatment at the bedside and be careful to avoid saying things which may distress the patient. Do not, for example, mention post-mortems. When it is apparent that something which the patient has heard has upset him you should find time to go back quietly afterwards to comfort and reassure him. It is a usual and good habit to have some clinical discussions away from the bed, in the corridor or elsewhere. It is also better not to mention the cost of drugs and treatment at the bedside for this may make the patient wonder whether he is to be denied some treatment because it is costly.

THE NIGHT ROUND

A regular visit at night should always be made to every acutely ill patient. Not only does it reassure him but gives confidence to the night nurse who may often be young and inexperienced and perhaps worried by her responsibilities.

FAILURE OF COMMUNICATION

This is a main source of the problems which arise in hospital. Illness is a shock to most patients and they have worries about the non-medical aspects of their stay in hospital. You should learn to appreciate the social and emotional aspects of illness and see that patients are fully informed about what is going on. You will find that the ward sister and medical social worker are skilled in doing this.

Failure to communicate is common too between doctors themselves and between doctors and nurses. Some examples of this are: failure to tell the nursing staff that a patient is to have a gastroscopy or an anaesthetic so that he arrives in the theatre with food in his stomach; failure to tell your surgical colleague after transferring a patient to his ward about drugs like insulin and steroids which the patient needs; failure to note the time of necropsy so that you miss it and failure to tell the laboratory that blood need no longer be kept because the patient has died.

If a patient moves to another ward *all* his papers and X-ray films should go with him.

Cultivate good telephone manners and be thoughtful about how you use this convenient but sometimes annoying instrument. It is best not to make complicated requests by phone until you have established good relations by personal contact. Some drug names sound alike so avoid phoning about them if possible. If you have to phone your chief try to learn when not to do it. He may take forty winks after lunch. No patient, however, must lack advice because of any reluctance to use the phone. If necessary you must do it but with apologies.

MEDICAL ETHICS AND ETIQUETTE

The fundamental principles of the relationship of doctors to their patients have always been the same. You will know instinctively what these principles are and how to apply them. There is no set of written rules though much has been written. (The BMA publishes a handbook on medical ethics.) To behave properly within an accepted code of etiquette depends on having or cultivating a sensitivity for the feelings of others and on considering how any contemplated action may affect one's colleagues. If etiquette is not observed the relationship between doctors becomes strained and the patient may suffer. The purpose of all we do is to benefit the patient. Etiquette furthers this end though the patient may sometimes feel it is designed for the doctor's rather than for his benefit. In hospital you work in a team and etiquette demands that one of the team is in charge. What the house physician does in his sphere of activity is all subject to the approval of his chief. You must only seek the opinion of a more senior person on another firm, if you can say that you do so on behalf of your chief.

Consultations may take place between housemen but any decision reached particularly if it involves alteration of treatment must be put to the consultant in charge.

When a patient is referred to another consultant for some special investigation he should be sent back afterwards and not taken over. Practice varies in this respect however and much depends on the consultants' personal knowledge of each other. You will find that most consultants have spheres in which they develop special interest. These should not be trespassed on. Do not borrow instruments (albeit hospital property) for example when they are for use in another's special sphere. The etiquette of prior request is nothing more than good manners.

If your patient or his relatives ask for a second opinion etiquette demands that you should take the request seriously and see that it goes to your chief. He will usually acquiesce to any such request and never pooh-pooh it. You may mention who is to pay any fee for it (the NHS if the consultation is at your request but the relatives if it is entirely theirs).

Your conscience
You must not allow matters concerning the patient's morals and your own religious beliefs and ethical standards to affect your clinical judgement. If you object on such grounds to assisting in operations such as abortions and vasectomies you should let your chief know in good time so that other arrangements can be made for assistance in carrying out the procedure he advises. On no account should you allow your personal feelings to interfere with what your chief decides is for the patient's welfare. In practice difficulties of this kind rarely arise. The job advertisement will not have mentioned abortions and the committee which appointed you will not have inquired about your

professional intentions about them unless your personal assistance would be necessary to maintain the service provided for by the Abortion Act 1968.

THE PATIENT WITH A FATAL DISEASE

Often the senses of a patient very ill from a fatal disease are dulled so that he does not ask questions, but sometimes a patient who thinks he is seriously ill will ask outright what is wrong with him and whether he will get better. If you cannot reassure him without hesitation it is best to hedge. Say there are a few more tests to be done or use some other device to put him off until you have had time to consider the question and to consult others. He may not ask again but when it is clear that he wants to be told and you know he is dying it is a good plan to see the relatives.

The clergyman should be brought if the patient wishes it and then it is often best to leave him to tell the patient.

In most cases you should assume that where there is life there is hope. It is a good rule to avoid telling the patient and particularly the young patient the hopeless truth, for as Sir Frederick Treves said, 'In the face of misfortune it is merciless to blot out hope.' It is your job to nourish hope as long as may be necessary. Often all you need to do is to lend a willing ear to the patient's lamentations. You will find that many patients are more concerned with their comfort than their salvation and so you should not say too much.

The relatives should be told the true position but with them also the blow must be softened. Before you give them bad news see that they are seated lest a sad situation becomes embarrassing. Warn them not to convey to the patient by word or attitude that hope has gone. Above all never let the seriously ill patient suspect that there is no more you can do for him.

After a patient's death many relatives appreciate a comforting talk with the doctor. They may be torturing themselves with guilty thoughts about some imaginary omission in their care of the lost one and perhaps wonder if, had they acted differently, all would have been well. It is kind to dispel such feelings and to explain that nothing they could have done would have altered the outcome.

THE NURSING STAFF AND THE SOCIAL AND ANCILLARY WORKERS

If you qualified overseas you may be confused by the different grades of nurses in British hospitals and by their dress. Ever since Florence

Nightingale prescribed special clothes for her nurses in the Crimea they have prided themselves on their uniforms, and patients have long been reassured by seeing 'splashes of scarlet and of lace'. Standard white uniforms for nurses are gradually being introduced but until they are fully in use considerable variety will persist. Many nurses wear a name and grade badge. Their grade may also be shown by coloured bands on their (usually paper) caps or, in the case of male nurses, by epaulettes. Nurses wearing the label 'post-basic' are fully trained and qualified but are having additional instruction in a special branch of nursing. Sisters' dresses are usually navy blue.

The present grades in the nursing profession resulted from the work of the Committee on Senior Nursing Staff Structure 1963 (the Salmon Report and its subsequent modifications). The effect has been to abolish the old post of Matron with her overall responsibility for all that happened in the nursing services of a hospital and to put in her place a nursing officer. The Matron's former housekeeping duties—linen, catering, cleaning etc. have been transferred to the appropriate functional manager who is not a nurse. A similar review took place in the community services.

The original 'Salmon' grades were given numbers, *e.g.* No. 6 for a ward sister, but these are rarely referred to now. Variations occur because of the size and numbers of hospitals in any given area but the chain of command from the Regional Health Authority downwards is as follows:

Regional Nursing Officer, the head of the nursing services of the Regional Health Authority.

Area Nursing Officer.

District Nursing Officer, the nurse who heads the nursing services of a District.

Divisional Nursing Officers for General Nursing, Midwifery and for Community Nursing.

Unit Nursing Officers. (In some districts there is a post of Senior Nursing Officer.)

Ward Sisters.

The DNO is in charge of all hospital and community nursing services including the former 'district nurses'. She is a member of the District Management Team and does not necessarily wear a uniform. Not every hospital has every grade of nurse and sometimes a nurse in one grade has to undertake duties, *e.g.* supervision of all surgical beds, which in another hospital would not be her responsibility.

In the wards and the departments all nurses wear uniform. The nurse in charge of a ward is a ward sister or, if male, a charge nurse.

They are addressed as Sister or Mr respectively. The next in command is the staff nurse, male or female. Many hospitals will have nurses in training. A *student* nurse trains for three years to become, after examination by the General Nursing Council, a State Registered Nurse (SRN). (Many hospitals still give their own certificates as they did before the examination for SRN was set up.) A *pupil* nurse trains for two years and then, on passing a less difficult examination, becomes a State Enrolled Nurse (SEN), sometimes referred to as a Qualified Practical Nurse. In general hospitals there are also Nursing Auxiliaries who receive some training, and Nursing Assistants in psychiatric hospitals for the mentally handicapped. They are all addressed as Nurse. Pre-nursing students (formerly called cadets) are young women under 18 who spend some time in the wards and departments and also go to a College of Education until they are old enough (18 years) to start their nursing training proper. In Scotland the equivalent of the SRN is the Registered General Nurse (RGN). Other non-statutory titles you may meet are ONC (Orthopaedic Nursing Certificate) and OND (Ophthalmic Nursing Diploma). Some nurses take a Diploma in Nursing and a few are graduate nurses with a university degree in nursing.

Your relationship to the nursing and ancillary staff
The ward is in the charge of Sister and all that goes on in it is her concern. Visitors and all who come to the ward, including yourself, do so with her permission. Although you can go to the ward virtually at any time it is courteous, if you have to do so at an unusual time, to express the hope that it will not be inconvenient. When Sister is off-duty the staff nurse is in charge and after her the next senior nurse. You should appreciate this chain of command and be sure that you speak to the right member of it. In your relations with the rest of the staff and particularly the ancillary staff a personal approach is best. It is amazing, for example, what the laboratory staff will do for the doctor who is *persona grata* and who goes to see them about what he wants. When you are better known to your colleagues a telephone conversation will often do instead.

Social workers
The three originally separately managed parts of the National Health Service (hospitals, general practice and Local Authority services) have been brought into line with the new local government structure. Members of the social services (formerly almoners), however, were not included in the new unified service and are now part of the social service department of the Local Authority. They are generally

addressed by name and do not wear a uniform but often have a name badge and white coat. They help patients with personal and domestic problems and arrange for such services as home helps and meals on wheels. Unlike the ancillary staff, social workers do not work under a doctor's direction but are nevertheless part of the multidisciplinary team which looks after your patients.

YOUR NEXT JOB

Unless you hold a rotating appointment you will have to seek your next job. *The Hospital Gazetteer* (4th edition, 1972, British Medical Association, price £3.50) will help you to choose where to apply.

The application. There will probably be many candidates and as your immediate object is to get on the short list for interview you should set out your *curriculum vitae* clearly. If there are blank periods between jobs state the reason for them. Always ask your referee's permission before using his name. Have the application and copies of testimonials typed and send them with a short hand-written covering letter. If your name is a long one and you sometimes abbreviate it you will avoid possible difficulties if you give your names in the unabbreviated form and in the same order and spelling on all the relevant documents. In preparation for an interview try to visit the hospital. If short-listed let the committee know you have taken the trouble to do this. Read the history of the hospital if there is one.

The interview. Make sure about travelling directions to guard against being late. If you cannot attend it is good manners to tell the committee. Being interviewed can be an ordeal if you are nervous. Try to look as if you are enjoying it. The chairman will put you at your ease and then invite members to ask questions in turn. Be ready for these. Remember that committee members are only human and so may be tired after interviewing many candidates so do not lapse into silence but speak up and keep the committee awake. Do not make them work hard to dig out the facts but do not on the other hand monopolise the conversation. You may expect some non-professional questions. At the end you may be invited to ask questions yourself and to emphasise any points which you feel have not been brought out. Let your own questions be brief and do not haggle about some point of detail. It gives a bad impression to ask about off-duty time at an interview, rather you should ask about how much experience you will get and say how keen you are to do the work. Job descriptions are now handed to all applicants and these should answer many of your questions.

When you move between non-resident posts do not worry about

removal expenses and legal fees. Ask The Area Health Authority for help with these or the Secretary of the BMA (if you are a member).

INTERNSHIPS IN FOREIGN COUNTRIES

Countries of the EEC

A doctor who is a citizen of any one of the nine countries of the European Economic Community ('Common Market') (Belgium, Denmark, France, Federal Republic of Germany, The Irish Republic, Italy, Luxembourg, The Netherlands and the United Kingdom) has had, from 1977, the right to practise in any of the other countries provided he can satisfy the authorities about his competence in its language. In France he will also have to pass an examination.

A special scheme still operates for those who wish to be interns in French hospitals. Forty-five posts in Paris and 13 in Lyon are offered annually. Applicants must be under 35, speak fluent French and have at least two years post-registration hospital experience. They must provide evidence of acceptance by a French teaching hospital in Paris or Lyon. Posts are for one year and the salary is 5500 F per month for Paris and 5000 F per month for Lyon. For Paris apply in French to Service Scientifique, Ambassade de France, 41 Parkside, Knightsbridge, London SW1X 7JP. For Lyon apply to Direction Générale des Hospices de Lyon, Service de Santé, 3 quai des Celestins, 69 Lyon, France.

USA

If your basic qualifications were not obtained in USA, Puerto Rico or Canada and you wish to work in an American hospital (but not in independent practice) you must be a fully registered practitioner and you will then have to pass the examination of The Educational Commission for Foreign Medical Graduates. This consists of a multiple choice paper on medicine and surgery and an English language proficiency test. It is held every January and July in Edinburgh, Liverpool and London and lasts one day. The cost is $100.00. Apply five months ahead to ECFMG, 3624 Market Street, Philadelphia, Pennsylvania 19104, USA. In addition, to obtain an entry visa to the United States as a member of the medical profession, you must pass the Visa Qualifying Examination and document your English language proficiency. The VQE lasts two days: first day, basic science; second day, clinical science. It is held once a year in September (in the UK in London only). The English language requirement is a qualification for the VQE and must be met prior to registration. The cost of the VQE is $200.00. Satisfactory results (both days) of the VQE are accepted for ECFMG certification in lieu of the official ECFMG examination. Exemptions are possible. You may be helped by the *ECFMG Examination Review* (3rd edn., 1972) published by the Medical Examination Publishing Co Inc., Flushing, New York. Casualty posts may be obtained through Medical Recruitment Services International Ltd, Box 2401, British Medical Journal.

The more senior posts are obtained through your medical school or privately but for a residency appointment you may answer an advertisement in the medical press or register with the National Intern and Resident Matching Program, 1603 Orrington Ave, Evanston, Illinois 60201, USA. Matching is made in March for posts starting in July.

The NIRMP is not a placement agency but a national clearing office for matching the preferences of students for internships and of interns for residencies with the hospitals' ratings of their applicants in order to assist students and interns in obtaining, to the extent possible, their choices of internships and residencies. Almost all approved US hospitals participate but they may appoint foreign medical graduates direct if they wish, provided that these candidates are not registered with the NIRMP. If you wish to register with the programme you must send in your Application Agreement together with the required $25 fee for receipt at the NIRMP office no later than September 30. The basic registration fee entitles you to list a maximum of 10 active choices or less on your rank order list. The NIRMP attempts to match you to the highest hospital on your list that has an opening for you. You get your first choice unless that hospital fills a post with an applicant it has ranked higher than you. When you are notified of your matching you are to sign a contract with that hospital.

The annual *AMA Directory of Accredited Residency Programs 1978-'79* is available for $ 4.50 plus $ 0.50 postage from The American Medical Association, Order Handling Unit, 535 North Dearborn Street, Chicago, Illinois 60610, USA.

Canada

To be an intern in Canada you must first fulfil the requirements of the immigration department and show evidence of an arranged position. Appropriate educational qualifications are required to satisfy the licensing authorities. These vary from province to province. Some have reciprocity with the GMC and others require the ECFMG certificate. You should therefore contact the licensing body of the province in which you wish to be an intern.

The Commonwealth and International Medical Advisory Bureau of The British Medical Association will give advice on posts overseas. It issues a leaflet on Contracts for Overseas Appointments.

Unemployment benefit
If you should find yourself in the unusual position of being genuinely unemployed and unable to obtain work of the kind you could properly expect to have, you can claim unemployment benefit provided you satisfy the contribution conditions. These are similar to those required for sickness benefit (*p* 24). You should apply to the local office of the Department of Employment and Productivity and seek inclusion on its Professional and Executive Register.

DISCLOSURE OF INFORMATION

Routine disclosure
A decision to pass on information from a patient's records especially if to a colleague will not be a problem when it is routinely accepted as being correct and done with implied consent. But if a request for information appears to go beyond this then you should consider it with anxious care and seek the advice of your chief. At a plaintiff's request a court may order a defendant to produce medical records but they are normally only shown to the doctors.

Inquiries by relatives and friends
These normal inquiries about health and progress should always be answered with courtesy and patience in general, and if possible, reassuring terms.

Confidential inquiries
These are in quite a different category. No employer or member of a patient's family or solicitor or other person acting on the patient's behalf should be given any confidential information without the patient's written consent. To act otherwise, particularly in cases of pregnancy and venereal disease, would be to place yourself in a position of peril with regard to breach of professional secrecy. Only by meticulous observation of this rule can you avoid the risk of serious trouble. If detailed information is wanted for some specific purpose, either during the illness or afterwards, ask for the request in writing and also, obtain the patient's written consent to its disclosure. It is usual to give information to a spouse about the wife or husband but this might be inadvisable if a hostile relationship existed. You should then refuse to discuss a patient even with his or her spouse.

Press inquiries
You should think out beforehand your attitude to Press inquiries about patients so that you will not be taken unawares. The basic

principle should be that the patient is entitled to decide what is disclosed to the Press for his illness is a private matter and if he wishes secrecy every effort should be made to maintain this. Sometimes, however, a well-known person has let it be known to friends that he is going into hospital and your common sense will tell you that some information should be given when sought. Accident cases have often come to public knowledge by the time you see them and can hardly fail to attract Press inquiries. Be careful not to mention the victim's name until you know the relatives have been told. If this cannot reasonably be done you should make this clear to the Press. It is no part of your duty to report to the Press unasked. Many hospitals have a specially designated person to deal with Press inquiries and you will no doubt be glad to refer inquirers to him. If it falls to you to answer it is quite proper for you to ask Press, radio and television inquirers to show documentary evidence of accreditation or to give a phone number for checking. When a patient flatly refuses to give permission for a report to be made you must meet all inquiries with the formula 'no comment'. It is important at all times to maintain good personal relations with the Press. Do not show an obstructive attitude by refusing information without good reason. If you explain why details should not be published the Press will often be content to print only an edited version obtained from non-hospital sources.

Clergymen's requests
It is sometimes thought that a clergyman's request for urgent information about a patient must be complied with but this is not so. A clergyman or indeed any third party has no more right to information about a patient than anyone else. In every case disclosure should only be made when it would be in the interests of the patient and preferably with his consent.

Police inquiries
If you see as a patient someone who admits to being or whom you suspect of having been involved in some crime you may wonder whether you have any duty to report to the police. You have certainly no duty to report petty crimes. Serious crime such as murder is another matter for here you have a citizen's duty to the community. Between these extremes your action should depend on the dictates of your conscience. If you feel you must keep your knowledge confidential you will be in no danger provided you do not accept any reward for keeping silent. Misprision or concealment of a felony is no longer an offence in itself. (During a period of civil disturbance, however, the Government may make a regulation requiring, under penalty, anyone

including a doctor who knows of any wounding or harm from the use of any offensive weapon to inform the police or a member of HM forces.) You must, of course, be careful not to take any active step to assist a criminal to avoid detection or to escape as this would render you liable to be charged for assisting an offender. Anything you say in answer to police inquiries may be used later in court and so you should take care that your statements are accurate. If, as may unfortunately happen, an action on your part is questioned as allegedly criminal you are not obliged to answer. Unless a person is in custody he cannot be 'detained for questioning' against his will and if he assists the police he does so voluntarily.

You may be called on by the police and asked for evidence which might help in the arrest of an alleged criminal. Have you seen a patient with a cut hand or can you lead the police to a young woman who has just had an abortion? Even though the police can act 'on information received' without disclosing your name you should never allow yourself to be stampeded by the emergency atmosphere and 'official' environment into saying something you might later regret. If you do speak, however, and tell the truth you need not fear prosecution for you will be legally correct. But you may be ethically wrong and on this conflict between law and ethics you must make your own decision. If you can consult the person about whom information is sought and get his permission to disclose the facts you will clearly be in the right. But this would be difficult for what law-breaker would agree to disclosure? In other circumstances you would be wise to regard your knowledge as confidential and only to disclose it if refusal or failure to do so might be contrary to the public interest or might render you liable to be charged as an accessory.

You have neither the right nor the duty to assist the police if doing so would involve a breach of secrecy and you are advised not to disclose unasked any information about a patient. But this does not cover the situation when you are legally required to give information such as when asked by the police about an accident. Even information obtained solely through your doctor-patient relationship may be disclosed if you felt that failure might bring harm to an innocent third party or cause risk to the community.

CLINICAL PHOTOGRAPHY

In general, permission should be obtained to photograph any patient but as the opportunity is often fleeting there is no objection to taking a photograph of a child or an unconscious patient without it. Permission should be obtained later to use such photographs.

LETTERS TO THE FAMILY DOCTOR

Many hospitals give the discharged patient a brief note for his doctor on a special form stating the diagnosis and recommended treatment. A letter giving full details should follow as soon as possible and it may fall to you to write it. To do this well is an art which takes time to learn. If possible use paper which (folded not more than once) fits the 175 mm x 125 mm record envelope. Give all relevant dates and numbers but avoid slang and a telegraphic style. Make it clear what your chief's recommendations are. When you hand a letter to the patient to take to his doctor make sure there is no bad news in it (*see p 5*). Your letter should be short. Tell the doctor what he will want to know, what drugs are advised and how long you think the patient should be off work. Do not omit to send a letter if the patient dies. The family doctor wants to know what happened and you should save him the embarrassment of finding out from the relatives or the newspaper. Many doctors appreciate an interim letter about any patient who is in hospital a long time.

SALES REPRESENTATIVES

Most drug firms send their representatives to hospitals to talk to the doctors. You should treat them with respect for they are nearly all qualified pharmacists and well briefed. As a rule they prefer to see your chief but they also seek to interest all doctors in their products. You may be too busy to see them but if you do you must make it clear that you only prescribe drugs on behalf of your chief and you cannot undertake to try new ones without his consent or for some material albeit professional reward. In any case the impression gained by trying a drug on a few patients may be quite wrong and trials other than properly planned and controlled ones are to be deprecated. Do not be too easily captivated by glib sales talk. When told of a new preparation you should ask:

1. The approved name if any.
2. What existing products does it resemble in composition and action?
3. What are its side effects and toxic manifestations?
4. What does the Medicines Commission say about it?

Blunderbuss preparations are generally frowned upon and if a tablet has more than one ingredient you should find out why.

Although the patient does not now have to pay the full cost of his drugs you should have some idea of prices. You should avoid a proprietary preparation when there is an official one of the same composition.

PROFESSIONAL SECRECY WHEN IN COURT

The only form of absolute professional privilege recognised by law is the obligation of secrecy between lawyers and their clients. It is not *legally* recognised in the case of doctors and so you have an obligation to answer questions put to you in the witness box. It is quite proper, however, if you find yourself asked for information when you do not hold the patient's consent to disclose it, to appeal to to the judge nevertheless to take the *professional* rule of secrecy into consideration. You should do it when the question is asked and say to the judge, 'My lord, it would involve a breach of professional secrecy if I were to answer this question. Am I compelled to answer?' You would then be wise to follow the judge's ruling though you could accept imprisonment for contempt of court instead if you still felt you could not answer. Sometimes a judge will allow information to be passed to him and counsel in the form of a note.

WHAT TO DO IN A CASE OF ALLEGED RAPE

While it is probable that many raped women make no complaint of it because they wish to escape court proceedings and the attendant notoriety an occasional victim may go at once to the police or her family doctor. Sometimes she may arrive at hospital and then it may fall to you to take the necessary action. Even so you would be wise to seek the help of a senior colleague. If you must obtain the evidence remember that you may have to disclose it in court later and so you should make notes at the time and keep them. There is no clear boundary between seduction and rape and in about 4 per cent of cases the problem will turn out to be rape fantasy. It may be preferable to exclude relatives and friends and let the woman tell you her own story but if she is very distressed it is helpful for a woman friend to stay with her. This presents no legal difficulty. Your questions should be the necessary ones to find out about the date of the last menstrual period and of the last intercourse, if any; the obstetrical and gynaecological history and whether on 'the pill'. It is not really your job to make a probing inquiry which is best left to the police. In any case the psychological aspects call for expert handling.

Since conclusive evidence soon disappears examine the woman in the lithotomy position when first seen and in a good light. Look for scratches and bruises and take charge of underclothing for examination for seminal stains. Note the state of and take a specimen of pubic hair. Look for bleeding and for bruising of the vagina and tearing of the hymen. There may be little or no damage to a woman accustomed to intercourse and more evidence is needed in such a case than in a frightened virgin who would be more likely to struggle. Try with a syringe to get some semen from the vagina. Its group may be helpful if it can be shown to differ from that of the blood of the alleged assailant. Make thin smears on new clean glass slides from any material aspirated. Put a high vaginal swab in transport medium for culture for gonococci. Take blood for a VDRL test (see p 202). Gonorrhoea cannot be detected less than a week after the rape and syphilis less than six so arrange for the woman to be seen in the VD clinic later by direct reference or via her family doctor. If she is unwilling to attend treat her prophylactically yourself by giving probenecid 1 g by mouth followed by ampicillin 3.5 g or preferably procaine penicillin BP 2.4 g i. m. into each buttock. If the possibility of pregnancy exists tell her of the courses she may take. She may wish for some action to terminate a possible pregnancy if the next period becomes overdue ('menstrual extraction').

Arrange to get the woman home where she should not be left unattended. Women victims of rape or sexual assault (recent or remote) can get sympathetic advice and a companion to accompany them to the doctor, police or court hearing from the Rape Crisis Centre PO Box 42, London N6 5BV (01-340 6913 from 1000 to 1800 hours; 01-340 6145 outside normal hours). The long-term psychosexual effects of rape, unless dealt with, may last for many years and wreck pre-existing relationships including marriage. The husband too may need referral for skilled help in coming to terms with the event. The victim's life-style may point to other problems such as drug addiction and homelessness.

If asked to examine a male accused of rape only do so with his full consent preferably written and witnessed. Tell him of his right to refuse. Look for scratches and bruises and examine the penis for recent turgescence and tears of the frenum. Make smears from any meatal moisture and take a specimen of pubic hair. Note signs of a struggle such as facial and genital scratches. Send blood for grouping.

HYSTERIA AND MALINGERING

This is a warning note about the malingerer and the hysteric with whom you may be faced in the Casualty Department and whose symptoms do not seem to you to be genuine. A high degree of suspicion is needed to avoid error.

A malingerer is 'one who is not ill and pretends that he is' in a deliberate attempt to deceive the doctor for a gainful purpose. Without the possibility of gain (usually financial) the diagnosis is very doubtful. The 'in' term for malingering is 'simulation' and this does not have an unpleasant connotation. Malingering may present as straightforward simulation of a disease not present or as exaggeration of a minor disability or as attribution of a disability to an injury which did not cause it. When it follows an industrial injury the symptoms are inversely proportional to the severity of the injury. You may feel confident that you have never been fooled by a malingerer but you can't say this because *ipso facto* if he succeeds in his act you won't know he was malingering. The malingerer complaining of pain is apt to show migratory localisation of its maximal site (Magnuson's test) whereas the site of 'real' pain is constant. Criminal malingering is less common than it was and it is unlikely to be met in the Casualty Department. But what is sometimes regarded as a chronic form called Münchausen's syndrome (*see p* 283) by Richard Asher is always being met. The patient tells a plausible story and may achieve admission and even submit to operation. Why he does this is a mystery for there seems to be no motive. The patient moves from one hospital to another not because he has been found out but rather, it seems, because of some kind of compulsive neurosis ('hospital addiction'). Sooner or later you will suspect that this story is false and when the patient sees that you have done so his behaviour may become offensive. It is unwise to attempt a diagnosis by confrontation for this rarely leads to confession. These 'perennial, peregrinating, problem patients' are sometimes described in the warning notices sent round to hospitals by the Regional Health Authority.

Hysteria is defined as 'the non-deliberate production of symptoms of illness to avoid an intolerable life situation'. It differs from malingering only in the degree to which the conscious mind participates in the picture. Even so, precise differentiation between conscious and unconscious simulation may be difficult. Some would restrict the term to 'conversion hysteria' meaning by this that an anxiety neurosis which has become intolerable is converted into loss of function. Others include in the term the 'hysterical personality'—a state of emotional immaturity previously included in the now obsolete term 'psychoneurosis'. The hysterical patient by contrast with the malingerer does not realise that he is producing the symptoms himself and is unconcerned about them. He will present in many ways—with loss of memory, loss of speech, loss of movement (paralysis), fits and even loss of consciousness. Make a careful inquiry and examination. You will then spot a flaw in the picture and will arrive at the correct conclusion that the condition does not have an organic basis. The flaw may be a flicker of the eyelids or a bit too much facial expression for an unconscious patient to have, or the ability to cough noisily though unable to talk. You must beware, however, of saying that a patient's symptoms are purely hysterical just because they are exaggerated. They may represent simply the 'functional overlay' superimposed on organic disease.

DRUNK?

In the absence of the police surgeon it may fall to you to meet a police request to see a person alleged to be drunk when in charge of a motor vehicle. (Doctors are not usually required in other offences connected with drunkenness.) As the relatives may ask also you should be clear about who has called you. Although you may be accustomed to examine patients with only a nurse or a relative present it is quite proper in a case of drunkenness for the police to be present (in England and Wales but not in Scotland) during your examination. The accused's own doctor may be present too but it is best for him not to question his patient until after your examination. You should record the exact time of the accident, your examination and all other events. The questions facing you are: (1) Is he ill? (2) Is he drunk? (3) How drunk is he? If you decide that hospital treatment is necessary that is all you need say. If you give a statement to the police make it a non-committal one without a diagnosis or opinion. When the police wish to take a breath test of a person already at hospital they must tell you first. You can object to it if you feel it would be prejudicial to the accused's proper care. You could similarly object if a specimen of blood or urine was wanted or even if the police wanted to move the patient. While you should co-operate with the police you are not required to assist them in getting consent or obtaining specimens. Consent to any reasonable examination may be presumed if the patient is too drunk to give it but you could only take a specimen from such a patient if it was for the sole purpose of establishing a diagnosis.

Make an ordinary physical examination. When under the influence of alcohol the temperature is subnormal, the pulse rapid and bounding, the pupils dilated and sluggish and the tongue dry. Speech is slurred and the breath smells of alcohol. The patient may gesticulate wildly and break down emotionally. Hiccup and salivation are additional features. Then apply some special test such as walking along a chalked line, reading, writing and using a telephone directory. If the patient protests that he has taken little or no alcohol let him provide a specimen of urine for testing. Keep it in the refrigerator.

If you can't decide whether the patient is drunk or ill keep him in.

Remember Osler's epigram, 'Better admit a patient to hospital dead drunk than turn him away to be discharged from the jail dead but sober a bit later.'

'Sobering up'

When a head injury is suspected in a drunken patient it is helpful to hasten the removal of the effects of alcohol. Laevulose significantly increases the rate of metabolism of ethyl alcohol and so a safe 'sobering up' technique is to give 100 g of laevulose in 20 g/dl solution i.v. 'Sobering up' injections containing nikethamide and insulin are less desirable but frusemide (Lasix) by causing a diuresis will lessen cerebral oedema which is sometimes in part responsible for the clinical picture.

BROADCASTING   S O S   MESSAGES

The BBC (tel. 01-580 4468) will broadcast a message asking relatives to go to a sick person only if you certify that the patient is *dangerously ill*; that other means of communication have failed and that the full name of the person wanted is known. Messages will not be accepted after the patient has died.

THERMOMETER READINGS

The 'normal' Fahrenheit reading of 98.4° corresponds to 36.9° centigrade (Celsius). To convert °F to °C subtract 32 and multiply by 5/9. To convert °C to °F multiply by 9/5 and add 32.

Modern clinical thermometers are not marked with the time they should be kept in the mouth but simply as quick and slow acting. In all cases adequate time should be allowed—usually at least two minutes. You can avoid worry about whether the thermometer has been in the mouth long enough and so whether a reading is accurate by the simple device of using two thermometers with the mercury in one shaken down lower than in the other. If they both record the same temperature it is accurate. If they record different temperatures they have not been in long enough. The disposable Temtake device records the mouth temperature in 60 seconds or less. As taking the temperature by rectum is not always acceptable some units use the Uritemp bottle (Portex Ltd) which records the temperature of the urine as it is passed. Try to spare the nursing staff by not expecting routine temperature readings on every patient. Those with apyrexial illnesses may be omitted from the 'temperature round' unless their condition suggests otherwise.

You may meet a nurse who is unsure about how to use a thermometer properly. Make sure that she knows the importance of shaking the mercury down below the temperature scale so that the case of hypothermia (*i.e.* temperature below 32°C, 95°F) can be found when the mercury fails to reach the scale. In this case a wide range thermometer (25 – 40°C, 77 – 104°F) should be used.

WEIGHT

Weight gain after growth ceases is (apart from oedema) due to fat and so it is reasonable to regard the weight at age 20 to 25 as optimal. Ideal weight does not increase with age. Tables may be used to relate height and weight or a nomogram may be used. Perhaps a better guide for the control of obesity is the amount of subcutaneous fat as shown by skinfold calipers.

Height and weight conversion factors
(These are retained as elderly patients will still state their height and weight in feet and pounds)

To convert	Multiply by
Inches to centimetres (cm)	2.539
Inches to metres (m)	0.0254
Feet to metres (m)	0.3048
Pounds to kilogram(s) (kg)	0.4535
Kilogram(s) to pounds (lb)	2.2

Diets
Special diets are ordered through the dietitian. You can learn much from her about their application such as ensuring that a patient on a low protein diet for renal disease has a high (2000 to 3000) calorie intake to avoid breakdown of body protein. The following list will help you to make a good guess at the calorie value of meals.

Calorie value of some foods

(1 oz = 30 g. 1 fluid ounce or 2 tablespoonsful = 30 ml)

In the SI system energy is expressed in joules. A joule (J) is the work done by a force of 1 Newton (N) acting over 1 metre, i.e. 1 J × 1 Nm. 1 small calorie = 4.2 J. Hence a 3000 calorie diet provides 12.6 mega joules (MJ).

High	g	Calories
Potato crisps	30	159
Chipped potatoes	180	410

Calorie value of some foods (*cont.*)

High	g	Calories
Fatty meat	60	190
Fairly lean meat	60	150
Fried plaice	180	390
2 Fried sausages, beef	120	324
2 Fried sausages, pork	150	372
Kipper	180	340
Herring, fried	150	200
Salmon, fresh	150	170
Salmon, tinned	150	120
Suet pudding	120	400
Roast potatoes	180	210
Bread, 3 slices	150	280
Butter and margarine	30	230
Bacon, fried	60	240 to 330
Sausage roll	60	260
Sponge cake	60	240
Fruit tart	120	240
Fruit cake	60	220
Mince pie	one	200
Macaroni, cooked	120	130
Honey	30	82
Biscuits, water 3	30	126
Biscuits, sweet 3	30	158
Chocolate, plain	30	155
Chocolate, milk	30	167
Ice cream	1 small tub	120

Moderate	g	Calories
Meat, very lean	60	128
Chicken	60	110
Steamed fish	120	110
Cheddar cheese	30	120
Boiled potatoes	180	200
Breakfast cereal	30	100
All Bran	30	88
Sardines in oil	30	85
Sardines in tomato	30	50
Blancmange	60	70
Milk	150 ml	130
Yoghurt	210 ml (one pot)	
full fat		125
low fat		94
fruit		175

Low	g	Calories
Egg	60 (= 1 egg)	90
Jelly	120	90
Grapes	120	90
Banana	120	80
Tinned fruit	120	100
Apple	120	50
Orange	120	40

Calorie value of some foods *(cont.)*

High	g	Calories
Broad beans	60	25
Baked beans	60	50
Peas	60	30
Beetroot	60	25
Sprouts	120	20
Carrots	60	10
Cabbage	120	10
Tomato	60	8
Lettuce	60	6
French beans	60	4
Marrow	60	4

Drinks		Calories
Beer- 300 ml		90
Spirits 70% proof. Calories per 30 ml		63
Sherry per glass 30 ml		
	dry	100
	sweet	115
Tea and coffee		nil
Milk 30 ml		20
Sugar 10 mg		40

POST-OPERATIVE ILLNESS

You may be approached by your surgical colleague about a patient in whom something has gone wrong after operation. It often means a consultation between the physician and surgeon concerned but you should be aware of the possibilities so as to be able to give your chief a true picture and collect the evidence he will want. However reassuring the house surgeon is about what his chief did, always consider whether something has gone wrong surgically. If it is not surgical the following list of possible complications may help.

Chest pain
Myocardial infarction
Pulmonary embolism
Pneumothorax
Mediastinal emphysema
Diaphragmatic
  irritation

Dyspnoea
Collapse of a lung
Pulmonary aspiration
Pleural effusion
Fat embolism
Left ventricular failure

Hypotension and shock
Hypovolaemia
Hyponatraemia
Cardiogenic shock
Septicaemia
Endocrine failure
Postoperative bleeding
Collapse following corticosteroid therapy

Hypertension
Phaeochromocytoma
Thyrotoxicosis
Fluid overload
Pre-eclampsia

Fluid and electrolyte disturbance
Potassium depletion
Potassium excess
Sodium depletion
Water depletion
Hypomagnesaemia

Abdominal and back pain
Acute porphyria
Addisonian crisis
Pancreatitis
Pylonephritis
Diabetic ketosis
Acute dilatation of the stomach
Paralytic ileus

Coma
Diabetic ketosis
Hypoglycaemia
Hypothyroidism
Hepatocellular failure
Electrolyte imbalance

Convulsions

Paresis and tetany

Hypothermia and pyrexia

Venous thrombosis
A loose non-occlusive thrombus may not cause leg signs (the 'silent leg syndrome') but is liable to embolise.
(An occasional pitfall in diagnosis is rupture of a Baker's cyst with leakage into the calf causing tenderness and Homans' sign. Knee arthrography with Hypaque will show the leak.)

INFECTIOUS DISEASES IN GENERAL WARDS

What should the house physician do when an infectious fever occurs in a general ward? There is no rule of thumb plan about isolation and quarantine. Our aim should be to prevent spread of the disease to susceptible patients and, at the same time, not to interrupt the work of the ward unnecessarily. Surveillance often achieves this object better than quarantine, but the nursing staff should be told what to look for, *e.g.* slight coryza and rise of temperature. Chickenpox and mumps can be regarded as almost inevitable and it is a good thing if healthy children can get over them before they grow up. Elaborate measures to escape them are not to be encouraged except in special cases. Any members of the staff who have not had the disease in question or have not been vaccinated against it should be carefully watched. It is best to let them leave the children's or maternity ward for an adult ward.

Although erysipelas, meningitis and poliomyelitis are of low infectivity it is usually best to transfer patients from general wards to the infectious diseases unit. If this is impossible barrier nursing should be used.

In the case of certain diseases the Medical Officer for Environmental

Health must be notified. In some areas he wishes to know about rubella also and other diseases may be made notifiable in special circumstances. The action to be taken in the ward is indicated in Table 1.

Table 1 Policy for infectious fevers in general wards

	Disposal of patients	Immunisation of contacts	Admissions	Disinfection
Amoebic dysentery	O	O	O	D
Anthrax	R	O	O	D
Bacillary dysentery	H	O	R	D
Chickenpox	H	O	R	D
Cholera	R	O	O	D
Diphtheria	R	P + A 1	O	D
Encephalitis	R	O	O	D
Enteric fever (typhoid & paratyphoid	R	O	O	D
Epidemic pleurodynia (Bornholm disease)	R	O	O	D
Erysipelas	H	O	O	D
Food poisoning	R	O	O	D
Gastroenteritis	R	O	O	D
Herpes simplex	H	O	O	D
Herpes zoster	H	O	O	D
Impetigo	H	O	O	D
Infective hepatitis (virus A & B)	R	O (? P)	O	D
Leprosy	S	O	O	D
Measles	H	O (? P)	O	D
Meningitis				
aseptic	R	O	O	D
meningococcal	R	O 2	O	D
pneumococcal	O or R	O	O	O
tuberculous	O or R	O or A	O	O
Mumps	H	O	O	D
Mycoplasma pneumonia	R	O	O	D
Paratyphoid (see Enteric)				
Poliomyelitis	R	A	O	D
Psittacosis	R	O	O	D
Q fever	R	O	O	D
Roseola infantum	H	O	O	O
Rubella	H	O	O	D
Salmonella infections	H	O	O	D
Scarlet fever	R	O	O	D
Staphylococcal infections	H	O	O	D
Typhoid (see Enteric)	R	O	O	D
Vaccinia	R	O	O	D
Whooping cough	R	O	O	D

Key:
1, Send nose and throat swabs from staff and patients in the ward.
2, Prophylactic sulphonamides to close contacts for 24 hours.

Disposal of patients: O, = no action; R, = remove to infectious diseases unit H, = remove to infectious diseases unit or home as appropriate; S, = special procedure-notify disease consultant and community physician at once.

Immunisation of infectious contacts: O, = no action; A, = active immunisation; P, = passive immunisation. (Give human immunoglobulin i.m., not i.v.)

Admission policy: O, = no action; R, = restrict admission to immunes; S, = special precautions, no admissions or discharges.

Disinfection: O, = no action; D, = disinfect bed, mattress and bed table; S, = special precautions, destroy bedding.

Note
Living measles virus vaccine is effective within the first few days of the incubation period.
A history of chickenpox is doubtful if there are no pock marks anywhere.

Table 2 Incubation, infectivity and quarantine

	Incubation in days	Infectivity	Quarantine in days
Chickenpox	Extremes 10 to 16 Commonest 14	Until all scabs are off	21
Diphtheria	2 to 5	Until two consecutive nose and throat swabs are negative	7
Measles	10 to 15 Normally Koplik's spots on the 9th day and rash on the 12th day	14 days from the appearance of the rash, or, in mild attacks, until the end of clinical symptoms	21
Rubella	14 to 21	7 days from the appearance of the rash	21
Mumps	Extremes 10 to 28 Commonest 17	1 week after glands subside	28
Whooping cough	7 to 10	21 days or until all catarrh has gone	14

The current list for infectious diseases notifiable in England and Wales is:

Acute encephalitis
Acute meningitis
Acute poliomyelitis
Anthrax
Cholera
Diphtheria
Dysentery (amoebic or bacillary)
Encephalitis
Ebola fever
Infective jaundice
Lassa fever
Leprosy
Leptospirosis
Malaria
Marburg disease
Measles
Ophthalmia neonatorum
Paratyphoid fever
Plague
Rabies
Relapsing fever
Scarlet fever
Smallpox
Tetanus
Tuberculosis
Typhoid fever
Typhus
Whooping cough
Yellow fever

Notification is no longer required in England and Wales in the case of pneumonia, acute rheumatism, erysipelas, membranous croup and puerperal pyrexia.

IMPORTED TROPICAL DISEASES

Any of the international quarantinable diseases (smallpox, cholera, plague and yellow fever) will be reported to the port or airport doctor on the general health declaration. They all call for hospitalisation of the victims and surveillance of the passengers. But even despite screening procedures some sick immigrants will get by. Others may develop illness later and confront you in hospital. Especially if the patient is European his illness may catch you unawares. A geographical history is very important and you should always remember to ask Professor Maegraith's question: *Unde venis?* (Where have you been and when were you there?) For some diseases even the briefest touchdown abroad is significant. The traveller may forget to show the yellow warning card he was given on arrival at the airport. (He is at present not given one at other ports of entry.) The history may enable you to exclude some conditions. For example African trypanosomiasis (sleeping sickness) needs to be thought of only if the patient has been in an area of Africa between 15°N and 15°S. Other geographically confined infections are leishmaniasis (kala-azar and oriental sore) and schistosomiasis (bilharzia). Table 3 will help you in your suspicions.

Malaria

Malignant tertian (falciparum) malaria is potentially lethal because parasitised red blood cells block cerebral capillaries. It may not develop until up to four weeks after arrival here and so the pyrexia, which is not periodic in the early stages, may easily be attributed to 'flu'. If the patient has come from Central Africa don't indulge in diagnostic guesswork but make thick and thin blood films (*p* 132) or take 2 ml of blood in a sequestrene bottle and send if necessary to one of the addresses on *p* 67. Don't delay treatment, however, but give chloroquine 800 mg at once followed by 200 mg 8 hourly for three days. Malignant malaria is not a relapsing illness because no parasites persist in the liver but benign tertian malaria may be seen in Asian immigrants as a non-life-threatening relapsing fever.

Typhoid and paratyphoid

These should be thought of in any patient returning from abroad with pyrexia, abdominal pain and constipation.

Diarrhoea

When due to amoebiasis this presents as bloody diarrhoea or slight looseness without pyrexia resembling ulcerative colitis. Advice may be obtained from the pathologist, the Hospital for Tropical Diseases (*see p* 67).

Table 3 Geographical distribution of some serious communicable diseases which may affect travellers

Key:-
- | Indigenous disease absent
- ○ Indigenous disease uncommon
- ◉ Indigenous disease common in some areas
- ● Indigenous disease widespread

Disease	Tropical Africa (West, Central and East)	Ethiopia	Southern Arabia and Yemen	Southern India and Sri Lanka	East Indies and Far East	Vietnam	Northern Australia	Pacific Islands	Central America	Caribbean Islands	Tropical South America	Northern Europe	Southern Europe	North Africa	South Africa	Egypt and the Middle East	Pakistan and Northern India	Far East	Australia and New Zealand	North America	Temperate South America
Yellow Fever	○	○	|	|	|	|	|	|	○	○	○	|	|	|	|	|	|	|	|	|	|
Typhus	◉	●	◉	○	●	◉	◉	◉	◉	◉	◉	○	○	○	○	◉	◉	●	○	○	○
Typhoid Fever	●	●	●	●	●	●	●	●	●	●	●	○	●	●	●	●	●	●	○	○	●
Trypanosomiasis	◉	|	|	|	|	|	|	|	◉	|	◉	|	|	|	|	|	|	|	|	|	|
Smallpox	●	●	|	●	●	|	|	|	|	|	●	|	|	|	◉	|	●	|	|	|	|
Schistosomiasis	●	●	●	|	◉	|	|	|	○	◉	●	|	○	◉	◉	●	○	◉	|	|	|
Relapsing Fever	○	◉	○	○	|	|	|	|	○	|	○	|	○	○	○	○	◉	○	|	○	○
Rabies	○	○	○	○	○	○	|	|	○	○	○	○	○	○	○	○	◉	○	|	○	○
Poliomyelitis	●	◉	◉	●	●	○	○	●	◉	●		○	◉	◉	◉	◉	●	○	○	○	◉
Plague	○	○	○	○	○	◉	|	|	○	|	◉	|	|	|	○	○	○	○	|	○	|
Malaria	●	◉	◉	●	●	◉	◉	◉	◉	●		|	|	◉	○	◉	◉	○	|	|	|
Leishmaniasis	○	○	○	○	◉	◉	|	|	◉	○	●	|	○	○	|	◉	◉	○	|	|	|
Dysentery	●	●	●	●	●	●	●	●	●	●		◉	◉	◉	◉	●	●	◉	◉	◉	◉
Cholera	|	|	|	◉	◉	◉	|	|	|	|		|	|	|	|	◉	|	|	|		
Amoebiasis	●	●	●	●	●	●	●	●	●	●		○	◉	○	◉	●	●	◉	○	○	◉

Regions within the Tropics: Tropical Africa (West, Central and East); Ethiopia; Southern Arabia and Yemen; Southern India and Sri Lanka; East Indies and Far East; Vietnam; Northern Australia; Pacific Islands; Central America; Caribbean Islands; Tropical South America

Regions outside the tropics: Northern Europe; Southern Europe; North Africa; South Africa; Egypt and the Middle East; Pakistan and Northern India; Far East; Australia and New Zealand; North America; Temperate South America

(From *Communicable Diseases Contracted Outside Great Britain* reproduced by kind permission of the controller of Her Majesty's Stationery Office)

Schistosomiasis (Bilharzia)

If this is suspected pool terminal specimens of urine over 24 hours and send to the laboratory. The container need not be sterilised.

Lassa fever

This may be imported and should be suspected if a person from West Africa has a toxic pyrexia and membranous pharyngitis. It is highly contagious and has a mortality of 50 per cent. The London School of Tropical Medicine should be contacted for convalescent serum. Admission should only be to a unit possessing high risk accommodation.

Other conditions to be watched for are leprosy, filariasis, trachoma and infestation by hook worms (ankylostomiasis) and the common round worm. Some non-tropical diseases now rare in Britain still persist abroad (*e.g.* diphtheria in Cyprus) and so may be encountered here. Lastly don't forget that a pyrexial Afro-Asian whose blood is negative for malaria is often found to have pulmonary tuberculosis.

Where to get advice on tropical diseases

London

The Hospital for Tropical Diseases, 4 St Pancras Way, London NW1 OPE (tel. 01-387 4411).
The London School of Hygiene and Tropical Medicine, Keppel Street, London WC1E 7HT (tel. 01-636 3041: ext. 201 -Epidemiological matters; ext 344 or 342—Malaria).

Liverpool

The Liverpool School of Tropical Medicine, Pembroke Place, Liverpool L3 5QA (tel. 051-709 7611).

Birmingham

Department of Communicable and Tropical Diseases, East Birmingham Hospital, Bordesley Green East, Birmingham B9 5ST (tel. 021-772 4311).

Immigrants and persons on long-term visits from overseas are a different problem. They may have any cosmopolitan disease but also a tropical disorder presenting as an emergency such as the crisis of sickle cell anaemia. Specialised advice can be obtained from the tropical disease units in Liverpool, London and Birmingham (*see above*).

Table 4a Percentile chart for boys

Age	Weight (kg)			Height (cm)			Skull circumference (cm)		
	3	50	97	3	50	97	3	50	97
Birth	2.5	3.5	4.4	–	50	–	30	35	38
3 m	4.4	5.7	7.2	55	60	65	38	41	43
6 m	6.2	7.8	9.8	62	66.5	71	41	44	46
9 m	7.6	9.3	11.6	66.5	71	76	43	46	47
12 m	8.4	10.3	12.8	70	75	80	45	47	49
18 m	9.4	11.7	14.2	75	81	87	46	49	51
2 yrs	10.2	12.7	15.7	80	87	93	47	50	52
3 yrs	11.6	14.7	17.8	86	95	102	48	50	53
4 yrs	13	15	21	94	101	110			
5 yrs	14	19	23	100	108	117	49	51	54
6 yrs	16	21	27	105	114	124			
7 yrs	17	23	30	110	120	130			
8 yrs	19	25	34	115	126	137	50	52	55
9 yrs	21	27.5	39	120	132	143			
10 yrs	23	30	44	125	137	148			
11 yrs	25	34	50	129	142	154			
12 yrs	27	38	58	133	147	160	51	54	56
13 yrs	30	43	64	138	153	168			
14 yrs	33	49	71	144	160	176	53	56	58
15 yrs	39	55	76	152	167	182			
16 yrs	46	60	79	158	172	185			
17 yrs	49	62	80	162	174	187			
18 yrs	50	64	82	162	175	187			

Table 4b Percentile chart for girls

Age	Weight (kg)			Height (cm)			Skull circumference (cm)		
	3	50	97	3	50	97	3	50	97
Birth	2.5	3.5	4.4	–	50	–	30	35	39
3 m	4.2	5.2	7.0	55	58	62	37	40	43
6 m	5.9	7.3	9.4	61	65	69	40	43	45
9 m	7.0	8.7	10.9	65	70	74	42	44	47
12 m	7.6	9.6	12.0	69	74	78	43	46	48
18 m	8.8	10.9	13.6	75	80	85	45	47	50
2 yrs	9.6	12.0	14.9	79	85	91	46	48	51
3 yrs	11.2	14.1	17.4	86	93	100	47	49	52
4 yrs	13	16	20	92	100	109			
5 yrs	15	18	23	98	107	116	48	50	53
6 yrs	16	20	27	104	114	123			
7 yrs	18	23	30	109	120	130			
8 yrs	19	25	35	114	125	136	50	52	54
9 yrs	21	28	40	120	130	142			
10 yrs	23	31	48	125	136	148			
11 yrs	25	35	56	130	143	155			
12 yrs	28	40	64	135	149	164	51	53	56
13 yrs	32	46	70	142	156	168			
14 yrs	37	51	73	148	160	172	52	54	57
15 yrs	42	54	74	150	162	173			
16 yrs	45	56	75	151	162	174			
17 yrs	46	56	75						
18 yrs	46	57	75						

INFANT DEVELOPMENT

Rate of increase of weight is 140g a week in the first 6 months and 90g a week in the second 6 months.

Teeth. Lower central incisors appear at 6 to 9 months. All milk teeth (20) are present at 2½ years. Permanent teeth (32) begin to appear at 6 years—(molars first) and all are erupted (except wisdoms) at 12 years.

Anterior fontanelle should be closed at 18 months.

Progress. An infant

Holds up his head	at 3 months
Sits propped up	at 6 months
Sits up alone	at 8 months
Crawls	at 9 months
Stands	at 12 months
Walks	at 12 to 15 months
Says words	at 1 year
Says sentences	at 2 years

Percentile charts for British boys and girls

It used to be assumed that the average or arithmetic means for heights and weights in the older tables were the normals but this is not so and it is indeed impossible to define the normal. The modern way of recording height, weight and other measurements is by the percentile chart. When a large series of measurements is arranged in increasing order the pth percentile is the value below which p% of the measurements fall. Growth charts generally have lines drawn on them representing the calculated 50th percentile or median and the third and 97th percentile. It should be noted that the 50th percentile or median is not the same as the arithmetic mean or average. Thus in the series 2 3 5 10 20 the mean is 8 but the median is 5.

When recording a child's height and weight we put down the actual figure and also the percentile. In using the chart if, for example, at the age of 5 years a child was on the 97th percentile for height and at 6 years he was on the 50th percentile when we would conclude that his growth had been retarded despite the fact that the weight was within what are regarded as normal limits. A child ought to travel up the same percentile as he grows. In practice growth and development charts are used but for reasons of space we print here as tables the relevant figures for three percentiles for the height, weight and skull circumference.

Infant feeding

This note is provided for the non-paediatric HP who may find himself faced with a problem of infant feeding. He will be wise to follow Sister's advice but should remind himself of the general principles.

The fluid requirements of an infant are 150 ml per kg body weight in each 24 hours (one-seventh of this on the first day, two-sevenths on the second day and so on).

The calorie requirements are 110 per kg in each 24 hours. The feeds should be based on the *expected* body weight for the age but the amount can only be reached gradually if the infant is much under-weight. The intervals between feeds should be between 3 and 5 hours so that the infant has 5 or 6 feeds in 24 hours more or less on demand.

The calorie value of both breast milk and most modified cow's milk preparations is 30 calories per 30 ml. From these simple facts the sufficiency of an infant's feeds can be easily calculated.

Breast feeding is for most babies superior to artificial feeding and therefore should be encouraged. If it should be necessary to feed a baby artificially then a cow's milk preparation modified to resemble breast milk i.e. with a low solute load should be used. Feeds must be carefully prepared according to the maker's instructions. They are mostly reconstituted 1 in 8 *i.e.* one measure of powder to 8 measures (30 ml) of water.

2

Clinical Procedures

URINE TESTING

Although taken over by the laboratory in many hospitals this dying art is really a clinical procedure to be performed on the ward by the doctor or nurse. When urine goes for laboratory tests send it as indicated in the test's requirements (*pp* 77, 133, 136, 138). When a 24 hour specimen is wanted warn the nursing staff against a common source of sampling error, namely failure to send the whole specimen but simply to fill a bottle. An even commoner error is for the nurse to send more than a 24 hour specimen because the urine passed on emptying the bladder at zero hour is not discarded but put into the bottle. No preservative need be added as a rule. Always be sure that the urine sent was passed by the patient in question. Sometimes ingenuity is needed to get a specimen and you may have to wring out a napkin or sheet. The Hollister self-adhesive U-Bag (Abbott Laboratories) enables urine to be easily collected from baby boys and girls into a plastic bag.

Reaction
Use a Universal Wide-range Indicator paper and compare the colour with the maker's card. It is better than litmus paper which is not very sensitive.

URINE TESTS

Protein ('albumin')

Albustix
(*Warning*. In performing this and all strip tests it is very important to follow carefully the directions on the leaflet in the pack. Faulty testing may give erroneous results. Make sure the strips are not out of date.)
   Dip (but do not leave) the strip in the urine. Protein produces a greenish-blue colour which should be compared with a colour chart. The + colour block corresponds to 10 mg albumin in 100 ml of urine.

A very alkaline urine may give a positive result, as will phenothiazine drugs and cetrimide. Bence Jones protein will also work the test but only in concentrations greater than 150 mg per dl. Traces of cetrimide give a blue colour.

Heat coagulation

Acidify the urine with a few drops of 20 per cent acetic acid and heat the upper part of the test tube in the flame. Resulting cloudiness is easily seen. The amount of protein in the urine is best determined in the laboratory but a rough estimate can be made from the heat test. A minimal cloud indicates about 10 mg per dl, a heavy cloud 300 mg per dl and a heavy coagulum 1000 mg per dl or more.

Reducing substances ('sugar')

Clinitest

Using the special dropper put five drops of urine in the clean dry test tube provided. After rinsing the dropper add 10 drops of water and then a Clinitest tablet. Do not shake. When boiling ceases a blue colour indicates a negative result. Any other colour is positive. The test can be used quantitatively by comparing the result with a colour chart (orange means 110 mmol/l (20 g/l) sugar). A transient orange colour which finally becomes greenish brown means more than 110 mmol/l (20 g/l) sugar. This 'orange flash' may be missed unless looked for. If only two drops of urine are used then an orange result means 275 mmol/l (50 g/l) of sugar ('two drop test'). Fructose, lactose and galactose give positive results. Ascorbic acid and the excretion products of nalidixic acid, aspirin, isoniazid and L-dopa can all act as reducing agents.

Clinistix

Dip the end of the strip in urine and tap off the excess. If it turns blue within 10 seconds glucose is present. This enzyme test is specific for glucose but as it is affected by changes in pH it is not quantitative. It is sensitive to quantities greater than 5.5 mmol/l (1 g/l). Vitamin C reduces the sensitivity and high levels can abolish it. This test fails to detect galactose and if congenital galactosaemia is suspected in infants the Clinitest must be used.

The Clinitest detects a minimum of about 14 mmol/l (2.5 g/l) of glucose. The enzyme test is more sensitive. Clinistix positive but Clinitest negative means that because of varying sensitivities the glucose concentration is between 5.5 and 14 mmol/l.

Diastix

This is a semi-quantitative strip test for glucose. The end of the strip is dipped in urine and the excess shaken off. The colour reaction is timed for precisely 30 seconds and then the developed colour compared against the colour blocks on the bottle label. These represent concentrations of glucose in urine of 5.5 (trace), 14 (+), 28 (++), 55 (+++) 111 mmol/l of urine.

Caution. Diastix alone is not recommended when there is a likelihood of ketonuria. 'Moderate' to 'large' amounts of acetoacetic acid may depress the colour response of Diastix. A complementary test for ketones with either Keto-Diastix or Ketostix is then advised.

Ketostix

These strips react with acetoacetic acid and acetone in urine, serum and plasma and do not react with betahydroxybutyric acid. The reagent area detects as little as 0.5 to 1 mmol acetoacetic acid per litre of urine, serum or plasma. It is less sensitive to acetone. The result is read from the colour blocks as negative, small (+), moderate (++) or large (+++).

Ketones

These are often referred to as 'acetone' but this substance though it may occur in the breath is only present in traces in fresh urine. Seventy per cent of the ketones in the urine consist of hydroxybutyric acid for which we cannot test. The remaining 30 per cent is nearly all acetoacetic acid. This can be detected by the nitroprusside test in a dilution of 1 in 125 000 which is too sensitive for clinical use. It has been replaced by the similar but less sensitive Acetest tablets. If positive it indicates more than 1 mmol acetoacetic acid per litre. Place a tablet on a clean dry surface and put a drop of urine on it. Wait for 30 seconds. When positive the colour varies from lavender to deep blue. When negative the tablet simply becomes creamy from wetting.

Ferric chloride test

Add 10 g/dl ferric chloride solution in 2.0 mol/l HCl to 5 ml of urine drop by drop. Diacetic acid is shown by a plum red colour. Phosphates give a precipitate but this dissolves when excess of ferric chloride is added. If the result is doubtful do a control test on normal urine. Salicylates and phenothiazines give a purple colour. Prior boiling does not abolish the reaction if due to drugs but it will drive off volatile diacetic acid and render subsequent tests negative.

Blood

Do not assume that because the test for protein is negative that blood must be absent. The amount of protein in enough blood to cause clinical haematuria will hardly show in the test for protein. Microscopy is a satisfactory test for blood in urine but 66 000 cells per ml must be present before detection is possible. Failing this and also if numerous pus cells make detection difficult a chemical test is necessary for free haemoglobin. Hemastix strips and also strips for combined tests (Hema-Combistix, Labstix and N-Multistix) are available. A blue colour in 30 seconds indicates the presence of blood. The Peroheme 40 (BDH Chemicals) test for blood in faeces can be used also for urine.

Bilirubin

Ictotest tablets
Bilirubin makes urine greenish brown and gives a stable yellow froth on shaking. Moisten an Ictotest mat with five drops of fresh urine and then put on it an Ictotest tablet. Place one drop of water on the tablet and a few seconds later another drop which washes fluid on to the mat. When bilirubin is present the mat around the tablet turns bluish-purple within 30 seconds. A slight pink colour after 30 seconds is negative. Drugs do not upset this test.

A semi-quantitative test for bilirubin is available on multiple test strips such as Labstix and N-Multistix. A brown colour indicates a positive reaction. It is less sensitive than the Ictotest.

Urobilinogen

Add 1 ml of Ehrlich's reagent (3 per cent *p*-dimethylamino-benzaldehyde in 50 per cent HC1) to 10 ml of fresh urine and allow to stand for five minutes. Urobilinogen and porphobilinogen both give a pink colour. Add 1 ml of saturated sodium acetate solution and 2 ml of chloroform. Shake for a minute. After settling, a pink colour in the lower (chloroform) layer means urobilinogen and the upper layer porphobilinogen. Sulphonamides, acetone and PAS interfere with these tests. The test is available in the form of Urobilistix strips which do not react with porphobilinogen in concentrations found in urine.

Urobilinogen is increased by hepatocellular damage and haemolytic diseases. It is absent in complete obstructive jaundice but may be present in excess when obstruction is incomplete.

TEST FOR BLOOD SUGAR

Dextrostix
Allow a large drop of blood to flow all over the reagent area on the

printed side of the strip. Wait 60 seconds exactly and wash off the blood with water from a wash bottle (the tap is too vigorous). Read the colour promptly. If positive it varies from grey to purple. Dextrostix results can be read visually between 1.4 mmol/l and 13.9 mmol/l. Semi-quantitative determinations up to 22.0 mmol/l can be obtained by reading Dextrostix in a reflectance colorimeter (Eyetone). (*Caution*. It is essential always to compare the unreacted Dextrostix strip against the 0 colour block. Discoloured strips must not be used.)

False high readings may be given if the drop of blood is contaminated by any alcohol-based cleaner applied to the skin.

CATHETERISATION

Warning
The indication is acute retention of urine. Urethral (as opposed to suprapubic) catheterisation should be avoided in chronic retention particularly if there is also overflow. Since bacteria are normally present in the distal urethra, it is impossible to catheterise in complete sterility, but, even so, secondary cystitis is rare after catheterisation except when there is residual urine. Catheterisation then ensures infection and often precipitates acute retention when the bladder refills. Never let a nurse persuade you to commit 'Foley folly' by catheterisation just to ensure a dry bed.

Sedation *see p* 81

Which catheter to use
Do not be appalled by the display of catheters which a surgeon has to choose from. A Foley catheter with a latex balloon is recommended and it is best to try a small one first. If, when it has to be removed, the balloon won't deflate, pass a ureteric catheter up the side channel to let the water off. It is dangerous to try to burst it by overdistension.

Technique of passage
Observe strict aseptic precautions and wear a mask. A catheter should preferably be used only once so choose one which is pre-sterilised and packed. Wash the penis with soap and water and then dab the meatus with 1 in 2000 chlorhexidine (Hibitane) solution. Isolate the area with sterile towels-preferably using one with a central hole for the penis. At this stage the operator should wash and put on sterile plastic gloves. Using the plastic nozzle of the tube of sterile jelly (1 g/dl lignocaine and 0.1 g/dl chlorhexidine (Hibitane) inject 10 ml into the urethra. (Warn the pathologist that you have done this if you send him a

specimen for poison tests.) Retain it by using a penile clamp for four to five minutes and massage some into the posterior urethra via the perineum—a towel intervening. Lubricate the catheter with the same jelly. Hold the penis between the finger and thumb of the left hand. Hold the catheter with the right hand and pass the tip into the urethra and then advance it as necessary. See that the part which is touched does not enter. If the catheter sticks, withdraw it a little and twist it round before trying again. Having entered the bladder, connect the catheter to a sterile, closed drainage bag.

Urine for microbiology
In males a midstream specimen should be passed straight into a wide-mouthed sterile container. It may be preferable to send the patient to the laboratory.

For women the following details of the 'clean catch' method should be explained by the nurse. Clean the vulva with moist swabs. Do not use any antiseptic and wash off soap thoroughly. Dry well with a clean towel. Remove the cap of the sterile container and put it down *rim upwards*. Be careful not to touch the inside of the container or cap. Take the container in one hand. Separate the labia with the fingers of the other hand. Start passing urine and allow some to fall into the pan. Stop for a moment and then hold the container in the stream. Replace the cap carefully, dry its outside and label it with your-name and date.

Catheterisation of women
Catheterisation should be avoided if at all possible. If other considerations make it necessary clean the labia majora by swabbing from before backwards with 1 in 2 000 chlorhexidine (Hibitane). Then separate the labia minora with the left thumb and index finger and clean with a swab. With a third swab clean the region of the meatus and leave this swab in place. Wash the hands again and then, hold the lubricated catheter near its tip, introduce it into the urethra. Urine flows immediately. Unless the meatus is clearly seen it is easy to make the mistake of passing the catheter into the vagina. A convenient outfit is the Alexa female speciment set (Henley Medical Supplies Ltd) consisting of a presterilised PVC catheter and collecting bag which is sealed after withdrawing the catheter.

Suprapubic puncture and catheterisation
This technique is necessary if you have to exclude with certainty any contamination of a urine specimen by urethral or vaginal organisms. It is used to solve problems such as repeated low bacterial counts and repeated obvious contamination in catheter specimens. It is essential

that the bladder is distended. If this cannot be confirmed by palpation and percussion give a drink and wait an hour or so until there is a strong urge to micturate. Prepare the suprapubic skin (see p 82). A local analgesic is not always needed but sedation (see p 81) may be advisable. A 9 cm 20 gauge needle on a Luer fitting 10 ml syringe is best but any long needle may be used. It should be entered in the midline 5 cm above the symphysis and directed downwards at an angle of about 30 degrees from the vertical. Ten ml of urine is sufficient for bacteriological examination. If a catheter is to be left in place for drainage a trocar and cannula can be used the catheter being passed down the cannula. It is better to use a special Argyle Ingram trocar catheter.

'PUT OUT YOUR TONGUE'

Many patients will expect you to practise this easiest of endoscopies and if you do it with a thoughtful look and cheerful grunt it can be reassuring. It can also be a diagnostic goldmine of useful information which cannot all be listed here. A few reminders may be acceptable. The smooth atropic teeth-indented tongue points to dietary deficiency (often iron and vitamin B_1) or bowel disease. Pigmentation should prompt search for it elsewhere and for associated symptoms, e.g. of Addison's disease. A dry tongue may point to general dehydration or the 'sicca syndrome' or drugs. Lastly tongue pain, ulceration, tremor and wasting may all be useful pointers to more generalised disorders. By daily practising tongue inspection you will build up a useful store of experience.

GASTRIC LAVAGE

This should only be done in a properly equipped room. It is not a bedside procedure. It carries the risk of aspiration of gastric contents. If this occurs immediate bronchoscopic suction is advisable. Failing this postural drainage should be tried. Hydrocortisone, penicillin and oxygen may all be needed. For indications and contraindications see p 266.

In the unconscious patient
Preliminary insertion of a cuffed endotracheal tube by an anaesthetist is essential. If, however, lavage is deemed necessary without this safeguard it must be done with the head low and the patient preferably prone over the end of a table. If an operating table is available the Trendelenburg position with the patient supine can be used. Some

prefer to have the patient in the left lateral position with the head low. Struggling is less likely in the prone position but the patient may have to be immobilised by straps or by wrapping him tightly in a blanket. Remove dentures and open the mouth with a gag or boxwood wedge with a central hole. Use a fairly stiff oesophageal tube preferably 3.75 m long and about 1 cm in diameter (for an adult) with several large holes cut into it near the end. Lubricate the tube and pass it through the hole in the wedge if this is used or over the tongue and quickly down the oesophagus. It is virtually impossible to enter the larynx. The end of the tube should be 50 cm from the incisor teeth in an adult and 25 cm in a child. It is an advantage to mark these distances on the tube by a safety pin in its wall (but not in its lumen). A Ryle's tube should not be used except when it is impossible to open the mouth. It could then be passed through the nose.

When the tube enters the stomach attach a Señorans's evacuator or large syringe and empty the stomach. In cases of poisoning the stomach contents and the first washings should be kept. Then attach a funnel and pour in warm water. Bicarbonate solution can be used but should be avoided in barbiturate poisoning. After about 300 ml of fluid have entered (less in children) but with the level of fluid still visible in it, lower the funnel over a pail on the floor and siphon off the fluid. A total amount of 10 litres should be used but the temptation to pour in a lot at a time should be resisted as this might force the pylorus and defeat the object of lavage.

In the conscious patient

This is a different proposition for the patient's consent must be obtained. He usually gives it. If he will not and you think his life would be in danger without it seek the advice of the Medical Social Worker in order to act under Section 29 of the Mental Health Act 1959.

Try to reassure the patient by explanation. Use the prone position and let somebody hold his hands. Hold the mouth open with a gag and proceed as in the unconscious patient. If the patient vomits there is danger of inhalation. Remove the tube (he will probably shoot it out anyway) and clear the pharynx by a sucker before reinserting the tube. Occasionally laryngeal spasm occurs. The tube should then be removed and reinserted when struggling has ceased.

In children

When in a conscious child gastric emptying is indicated but lavage cannot be accomplished give Ipecacuanha Paediatric Emetic Draught BPC 10 ml (for age 6 to 18 months) and 15 ml (for age 18 months to 5 years) followed by water. Repeat the dose in 20 minutes if vomiting does not ensue. Beware of ordering Ipecac Syrup USP as Ipecacuanha liquid extract may be mistaken for it and being concentrated is very toxic.

OESOPHAGEAL TAMPONADE

Test the trilumen Sengstaken-Blakemore tube for puncture of its balloons. Spray the pharynx with 2 g/dl lignocaine. With the patient on his left side pass the tube, lubricated with glycerine, into the stomach using firm pressure. When the end is in the stomach inject 120 to 150 ml of water containing about 10 per cent of Hypaque into the gastric balloon. Pull on the tube to engage the gastric balloon in the cardia and tape its end to the face. (It is inadvisable to apply traction to the tube as formerly advocated.) If the patient is not bleeding at the time the

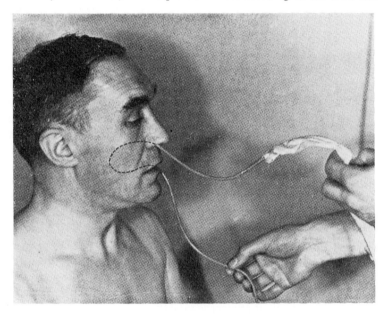

Fig. 1 Use of Ryle's tube to facilitate passage of balloon through the nose.

position of the tube may be checked radiologically. This step should be omitted if the patient is bleeding and the oesophageal balloon should be inflated to a pressure of 40 cm of water on the Tycos gauge. A Ryle's tube attached to the oesophageal tube allows for pharyngeal aspiration. The oesophageal balloon may be left inflated for two hours but should be let down for three minutes every hour. The tube may be used for periods of up to 48 hours but after this there is a risk of pressure necrosis of the oesophageal muscosa. Gastric aspiration should be used between feeds given down the tube. A soft rubber disposable tube may be introduced through the nose using an attached Ryle's tube to facilitate passage (Fig. 1). The chief risk is laryngeal obstruction from upward displacement of the tube. If this occurs deflate at once and if necessary cut the tube across.

THE USE OF SYRINGES

The house physician should carefully avoid bad syringe habits.

1. Before using a needle on a patient always see that he is sitting or lying down.

2. Always use 'once only' needles.

3. When taking blood see that the vein is prominent and the patient relaxed. Always use a dry syringe and needle. The prolonged use of a tourniquet and excessive forearm exercise must be avoided for it may cause false electrolyte values especially of potassium. Test to see that the piston will move freely.

4. Avoid unnecessary venepuncture by taking sufficient blood for all your tests.

5. Always detach the needle before expelling blood. Otherwise some haemolysis results.

6. Use disposable syringes. If others must be used dismantle and wash them immediately after use. This will avoid the embarrassment of a stuck piston.

7. Have a spare syringe at hand in case you drop one.

8. Beware of 'blind' venepuncture in a haemophilic. Consult your chief.

9. Avoid inadvertent i.v. injection by forming the habit of pulling back the piston to show that the needle is not is a blood vessel.

10. Read the label on the ampoule as well as on the box. Test to see that the piston will move easily but start venepuncture with the piston fully depressed to avoid a bubble.

SEDATION FOR MINOR PROCEDURES

Valium (diazepam) 20 mg i.v. via a winged needle in a forearm vein is a suitable dose for an adult who is not taking other sedatives. Give about 2.5 mg per minute until drooping of the eyelids and slurring of speech tell you that you can proceed. As it is not an analgesic it may be preceded by pentazocine (Fortral) 30 mg i.v. Oxygen and naloxone (Narcan) should be at hand in case there is respiratory depression. A outpatient should be kept for a few hours and not allowed home unless accompanied. This technique is not suitable for children for whom Vallergan (trimeprazine) syrup 2 to 4 mg per kg by mouth is recommended.

SKIN PREPARATION

Although injection through the unprepared skin is often done with impunity by diabetics it is wiser for the doctor to prepare the skin before any needling. A dab with a Mediswab (70 per cent w/w isopropyl alcohol BP) or methylated spirit may be sufficient but a better method is to cleanse the area with acetone or spirit to remove the skin oils harbouring bacteria and then to apply Weak Solution of Iodine BP; remove this after 2 minutes with spirit (70 per cent w/w). Iodine must not be left under a sealed dressing. If there is a history of iodine sensitivity use chlorhexidine (Hibitane) instead.

INJECTIONS

Don't regard the minor procedure of giving an injection as hardly worthy of a doctor but aim at a perfect technique and the reputation

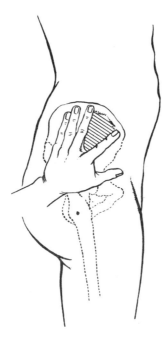

Fig. 2 Cross-hatched area between index and middle fingers shows where to give an i.m. injection into the buttock.

that your injections are painless. It is best to conform to the ritual of applying an antiseptic and to let the patient be aware of this. Intramuscular injections are generally not as painful as subcutaneous ones.

Subcutaneous injections

Use the smallest suitable needle. Don't jab it straight in. Let it rest on the skin for several seconds before you push it in. The idea is to separate the stimuli of touch and pain so that the patient, being occupied with touch, is less sensitive to pain. A similar technique is to tell the patient he will feel pressure and then to press on the site with the finger before inserting the needle.

Intramuscular injections

These will usually be given by a nurse. The deltoid muscle will accommodate small injections but for large ones the midthigh (vastus externus) or buttock is best. In the buttock the upper and outer quadrant as near to the iliac crest as possible is advised, to avoid damage to the sciatic nerve. Place the index finger vertically (in a standing patient) with its tip on the anterior superior iliac spine. Abduct the middle finger (as in Sir Winston Churchill's V for Victory sign) and place its tip just below the iliac crest. The injection site lies within the triangle formed by these fingers and the iliac crest (Fig 2). (Reverse the position of the fingers when injecting the opposite buttock.)

Draw the skin and subcutaneous tissues aside (so that they break the needle track when they fall back). Apply suction to make sure a blood vessel has not been entered. After the injection leave the needle in place for a few seconds before withdrawal and then press on the site for a while.

Don't inject adrenaline i.m. or into the buttock, because of the risk of gas gangrene from local lowering of oxygen tension. Pain caused by injection of certain drugs can be greatly lessened by combining the drug with an equal volume of 2 g/dl lignocaine in the syringe.

VENEPUNCTURE

An antecubital vein is generally used for taking blood. The median one is best, being less mobile than the lateral one. As the patient may faint be sure, if he is not in bed, that he is comfortably seated. Never be tempted by very good veins to take blood by needle only i.e. without a syringe for you will get blood which may contain the virus of hepatitis on your finger. Choose a syringe larger than the volume of blood wanted to allow for air bubbles. A 10 ml syringe is best. Ordinary hand washing is sufficient provided the needle and nozzle are not touched.

Make sure the container for the specimen is ready and its cap loosened. Put on a sphygmomanometer cuff with its tubes away from the puncture site and inflate to 90–100 mmHg Alternatively use a Velcro strip or soft rubber tube tied round the arm for quick release. Don't let it pinch the skin. Ask to patient to make a fist. You can. use the antiseptic of your choice on the skin but do not let any trickle on the arm lest the patient thinks it is blood. Prepare the skin (*see p* 82). When blood is taken for alcohol estimation, however, only non-alcoholic cleansers must be used. Do not choose the smallest needle for it will make the flow slow and can cause haemolysis. It is best not to let the patient see the needle or to mention the word blood. A short bevel is preferable and less liable to transfix the vein. Immobilise the skin and steady the vein with the index finger before inserting the needle either directly or into the skin first and then the vein. Most doctors have the bevel upwards despite the theoretical advantage that the bevel downwards position is less likely to damage the opposite wall of the vein. The bevel could be turned to the down position after entry. Keep your eye on where the needle point is so that any extravasation can be seen at once. Apply gentle suction (if it is too great air will enter). When sufficient blood has been obtained release the tourniquet and tell the patient to unclench fist before removing the needle. Press a swab on the site and raise the arm. Detach the needle and fill and label the container. Put an adhesive dressing on the arm. The whole operation should not take long since prolonged venestasis will raise the calcium and potassium levels in the specimen.

Difficulties

'No veins'. Flick the skin with the finger and wrap the arm in a hot moist towel to make the veins dilate. Veins you can feel are better and those you can only see. The vein finder (Alpha laboratories) may be used.

Haematoma. If extravasation is seen release the tourniquet and try the other arm.

JUGULAR VENEPUNCTURE

(For technique in an infant *see p* 95).

The internal jugular vein is well suited for insertion of a central venous pressure catheter. Place the patient in Trendelenburg's position or with the head and thorax low (to avoid air embolism) and let him perform Valsalva's manoeuvre (to distend the vein). Turn the head to the opposite side. The entry point is 5 cm from the upper border of the clavicle at the posterior border of the sternomastoid muscle. Aim for the suprasternal notch. The vein being wide is easily entered, with a slight 'give'.

Another technique depends on the fact that the end of the jugular vein lies behind the clavicular head of the sternomastoid muscle. Define the triangle formed by the sternal and clavicular heads of the sternomastoid muscle and the inner end of the clavicle. Enter the needle at the apex of this triangle and direct it caudally and laterally towards the anterior end of the first rib behind the clavicle.

INTRAVENOUS INJECTIONS

Proceed as for venepuncture. Pull back the piston to show that you have entered the vein. Release the tourniquet and inject the drug slowly. If the blood you draw back is bright red it may mean that an artery has been entered. This rare accident can occur if there is an aberrant artery between the skin and the fascia and if pulsation in it has been abolished by a tight tourniquet. So palpate for pulsation first. If the solution to be injected is dark it is difficult to see blood enter the syringe and to note its colour. A glass adaptor as a sight chamber between the syringe and the needle is then a great help. If you realise that you have injected into an artery do not withdraw the needle but inject at once 5ml of 2 g/dl lignocaine and call a senior colleague.

Two drugs should not be given i.v. at the same time. It is a good plan to avoid giving a second drug until after the half life of the first. Ask the pharmacy what a drug's half life is.

INTRAVENOUS INFUSION

The many devices on the market may be classed as follows:-

1. Winged short needles with tubing attached.

2. Short cannulas made of various plastics including Teflon. The needle passes inside the cannula as in the Medicut. It allows easy insertion of a tube for i.v. feeding and also a cardiac pacing electrode. A local analgesic is advisable.

3. Indwelling radio-opaque catheters of varying lengths. Needle outside the catheter. Needle can be removed when catheter is in place. There is a risk of severing the catheter when it is removed. Needle and catheter should be removed together when necessary. A long catheter may be supplied in the form of a cartridge.

4. Cannulas for cut down. No needle.

Warning
Solutions for i.v. infusion are now often supplied in double plastic

bags, the outer one being for protection only. Examine in bright transmitted light and reject:

1. If the inner bag is damaged.
2. If the solution is not absolutely clear.
3. If there are visible droplets between the inner and outer bags.

Needle and cannula technique

An easily palpable and visible forearm vein may be used but the bend of the elbow should be avoided. Aim for a junction of veins because this is generally fixed. If a leg vein is used the best one is just anterior and proximal to the medial malleolus. Leg veins are prone to thrombosis, especially if varicose, and it is well to avoid them if possible or to put a little heparin in the infusion bottle. Shave and prepare the skin over the whole area where any strapping may be used. Put on a sphygmomanometer cuff with the rubber leads upwards and place a waterproof sheet under the arm to avoid soiling the bed. Then scrub up and dry the hands with a sterile towel or with spirit and a swab. Cover all parts except the site of operation with sterile towels. Infiltrate the site intradermally and subcutaneously with 2 g/dl lignocaine. Invert the drip bag and release the clip so that the tube fills with fluid and all air bubbles are removed. Squeeze the drip chamber so that it is about half full. Clip the tube with a haemostat near the adaptor on the end and hang it on the drip stand ready for use.

Subclavian venepuncture

The right infraclavicular approach is best for a right-handed operator as it avoids possible injury to the thoracic duct. First study the anatomy. The large subclavian vein arches over the first rib and lies immediately behind the middle third of the clavicle. Ideally subclavian venepuncture should be done under aseptic conditions in the surgical theatre.

Let the patient be supine with a 5 degree head-down tilt to avoid the risk of air embolism. Shave the skin carefully if necessary below the right clavicle and prepare it (*see p* 82). Infiltrate the area 1 cm below the mid-point of the clavicle with 2 g/l lignocaine. Make a 2 mm wide hole in the skin with a scalpel. Insert a 14 gauge Sherwood Argyle Medicut needle attached to a syringe (needle inside cannula). Advance the needle tip close to the underside of the clavicle but don't injure the periosteum as this would be painful. Apply suction as the needle is advanced. The vein should be easily entered, sometimes with a slight 'give'. There must be no poking about. After entering the vein alter the direction of the needle so that it aims at the sterno-clavicular joint.

This is to facilitate entry of the catheter into the subclavian vein and superior vena cava. Withdraw the needle and advance the catheter.

Cut-down technique

This is rarely needed these days but may be necessary if a vein is inaccessible through the skin.

After infiltration with 2 g/dl lignocaine make a 2.5 cm incision along or transversely across the vein and divide the superficial fascia. (Longitudinal cut-down incisions heal better than transverse ones in the leg; in the arm there is little difference.) Free 2.5 cm of vein by inserting closed sharp-pointed scissors or a small haemostat and opening the blades longitudinally. Free the vein similarly from its deeper attachments. Using an aneurysm needle draw a loop of ligature material (Dexon 3/0) under it and then by cutting the loop leave two ligatures *in situ*. Tie each loop loosely with a single knot and secure both ends of each piece by artery forceps. Hold the artery forceps between the middle, ring and little fingers respectively, so that the vein is held taut. Make a vertical nick in the vein with a small knife and relax the tension on the vein to see that blood flows. Insert the plastic cannula and connect the drip. If the vein is small it is an advantage to put a finger tip under it, so that the end of the cannula can be pressed against it. Tie the distal ligature to obliterate the vein and then the proximal one very securely round the cannula. Thread a needle to the ends of the ligature and bring it through the incision. The ligature may be tied over pieces of gauze or in the case of the distal ones around the flange of the cannula.

Causes of failure to flow

1. Failure to release the tourniquet.
2. Venous spasm. Pinch the tube with one hand and milk its contents towards the needle. Inject a few millilitres of 2 g/dl lignocaine. Place hot-water bottles on the arm.
3. Air inlet blocked.
4. Filter blocked with clot.
5. Kinked tubing.
6. Point of cannula against side of vein.
7. Clot in needle. Avoid this by connecting to drip quickly so as not to leave blood in the needle. Always keep the flow going continuously lest a little blood enters the cannula and clots in it.
8. Tight bandaging.

Drip chamber full of fluid

When the air column in the drip bulb is lost the rate of flow cannot be observed. Unhook and lower the container. Squeeze the contents of the drip chamber back into it. On raising the container there will be a fluid level in the drip chamber.

Rate of drip (see p 257)

Speeding the drip
This can be done by increasing the pressure in the bag by wrapping it in a sphygmomanometer cuff. Alternatively and preferably a rotatory peristaltic hand pump may be attached to the drip tubing.

Heparinisation
If infusion is intermittent the cannula should be flushed with heparin solution after each infusion. The Venflon device facilitates this. Use 2 ml of Heparin (Mucous) Injection BP (Hep-Rinse) 100 units per ml diluting if need be with isosmotic sodium chloride solution to keep the i.v. line patent.

Taking down the drip
This must be done carefully with proper closure of the wound. The ligatures under the vein may be removed after cutting down, so that its patency is maintained just as it is after needling. Simple pressure is applied and the skin sutured accurately.

Air embolism
This is the main urgent risk of i.v. infusion. To avoid it:

1. Don't use tubing which is loose, cracked or opaque and not emptied of air.
2. Don't let the level of fluid fall below the orifice of the exit tube. (A special drip indicator will give visual or audible warning of this.)
3. Don't apply positive pressure except under your own continuous supervision. The level of fluid must on no account be allowed to fall below the tip of the filter.
4. Put the clip near the vein rather than near the container.
5. Take a loop of tubing below the level of the vein.
6. Let the needle entry point be lower than the heart.

Intravenous infusion in babies
A scalp vein is usually convenient. Shave the scalp over the temple. Apply finger pressure in front of the ear. Three or four small veins will be seen. Flick them gently to make them stand out. An elastic band round the head is sometimes a help. A short winged needle with plastic tubing attached is preferred. After insertion the device can be fixed

with a plaster of Paris bandage. Because the amounts of infused fluid must be known exactly special measuring burettes must be used. The long saphenous vein at the ankle is also popular because it is large and anatomically constant.

ABDOMINAL PARACENTESIS

This is mainly done for diagnostic purposes now that diuretics have lessened the need for peritoneal drainage. Give a sedative if the patient is anxious, (see p 81). Make sure the bladder is empty. Prepare the skin (p 82). The favoured puncture sites are in right and left iliac fossae midway between the umbilicus and the anterior superior iliac spine or the right and left subcostal regions—all lateral to the rectus muscle. Avoid scarred areas, they may mean adherent bowel.

Prepare the skin (see p 82) and put on sterile towels. Inject 2 g/dl lignocaine into the skin and subcutaneously. Introduce a Medicut type needle (needle inside cannula). A polythene tube put in through a needle avoids the risk of bowel damage during drainage. If much fluid is easily obtained and you wonder whether it is urine, have the urea content estimated. Ascitic fluid contains about 5 mmol urea per litre whereas urine contains nearly 100 times as much.

Send 10 ml of fluid in a sequestrene tube for protein testing and a similar amount if amylase estimation is wanted. For cytology 100 ml with added citrate is needed. For culture send 20 ml in a sterile container. Consult the laboratory first. A large volume, citrated, is needed, if tuberculosis is suspected (see p 149).

PERITONEAL DRAINAGE

If this is desired prepare as for paracentesis but put on a many-tailed bandage first. Prepare the skin (see p 82), make a scalpel nick and push in the trocar and cannula. The best instrument (Willen Bros, 44 New Cavendish Street, London W1M 8HE) has a blunt-ended cannula with side holes: is of narrow bore (2 mm outside diameter); has a wide flange to allow easy fixation and is quickly connected to the drainage tube by a Luer-Lok. As fluid is removed the bandage should be tightened.

PERITONEAL BIOPSY

Prepare as for abdominal paracentesis. Use a Cope needle. Place this with its stylet into the cannula and introduce these into the peritoneal cavity. Remove the stilette and take a specimen of fluid. If no fluid can be obtained it is unwise to proceed. Replace the needle by the hooked biopsy trocar and turn this until it catches on the peritoneum. While maintaining traction advance the outer cannula so that its cutting edge removes some peritoneum. The advantage of this needle is that the inner cannula can be kept in position and further specimens obtained. An Abram's pleural biopsy needle (p 94) could be used but only one specimen would be obtained from each puncture.

PERITONEAL DIALYSIS

Indications
Peritoneal dialysis (PD) may be indicated in all types of acute and acute on chronic renal failure and occasionally to treat poisoning by dialysable agents. Its advantages are that the patient does not have to be bled, his veins remain untouched and there is no need for fluid and protein restriction. It is, however, about four times slower than haemodialysis and may prove technically impossible on account of ileus or adhesions. Relative contraindications are advanced pregnancy, large hernias, abdominal injury and recent surgery which has opened up the retroperitoneal space or disturbed the continuity of the peritoneum.

Dialysis fluid

The basic composition is:

Na	140.5 mmol/litre
Ca	1.75 mmol/litre
Mg	0.75 mmol/litre
Cl	101.0 mmol/litre
Lactate	44.5 mmol/litre
Dextrose	76 mmol/litre

As this solution contains no potassium it may be used for the treatment of hyperkalaemia. The potassium level should be reduced with caution in digitalised patients lest digitalis toxicity be precipitated. When removal of potassium is considered inadvisable a solution containing potassium chloride 3 to 4 mmol/litre should be used. Commercial solutions are generally supplied with two concentrations of sodium and two of dextrose in 1- or 10-litre containers. The high dextrose solution is used for the rapid removal of oedema fluid. Normally the low sodium fluid is recommended except in hypotensive patients. Heparin 1000 units per litre should be added to the first few exchanges to prevent occlusion of the cannula by fibrin. Gentamicin 4 to 6 mg per litre can be added but is best reserved for the treatment of established peritoneal infection. This is suggested by abdominal pain, tenderness, fever and a cloudy effluent and is confirmed by culture. Rarely monilial peritonitis ensues and is best treated by the addition of amphotericin B 1 mg per litre of dialysis fluid. Occasionally the same symptom complex is observed during PD from chemical peritonitis.

Apparatus
The plastic catheter of the Trocath (Chas. F. Thackray, Ltd) fits over a long stilette introducer which makes a trocar unnecessary. The puncture is slightly smaller than the catheter diameter and this ensures a tight fit and minimises leakage into the abdominal wall. Warming the bag of fluid to 40°C in a water bath makes for comfort and favours ionic exchanges.

Technique
Shave the skin of the lower abdomen but leave the pubic hair. Prepare the abdominal wall (*see p* 82), and place towels as for laparotomy. Let the patient empty his bladder or else catheterise him. Infiltrate 5 ml of 1 g/dl lignocaine down to the peritoneum in either iliac fossa and introduce 1.5 to 2.0 litres of warmed dialysis fluid through the anaesthetised area by means of a plastic i.v. type of needle (Medicut 16 gauge) and then withdraw the needle. Next choose a place in the midline one-third of the way from the umbilicus to the symphysis but avoid any scars. Infiltrate down to the linea alba with 1 g/dl lignocaine. Nick the skin with a small scalpel and pass it down till it grates on the linea alba. There will be very little bleeding in the midline. The Trocath is more easily inserted with the abdominal muscles contracted, so ask the patient to take a deep breath and raise his shoulders off the bed. Considerable force is needed to insert the Trocath. A 'give' indicates that it has entered the peritoneal space. Withdraw the stilette 4 cm and gently advance the catheter aiming for the true pelvis. If it meets resistance withdraw slightly and change the direction. It is normal for some fluid to come up the catheter even when the preliminary injection into the iliac fossa has been omitted. All the fenestrations of the catheter must be within the peritoneal space. Trim all but 4 cm of the projecting catheter. Securing of the catheter and the metal disc by adhesive is best delayed until a free flow is established. When fixing the fluid line to the chest or thigh this should be separate from the abdominal gamgee and Elastoplast dressing to avoid accidental drag on the cannula. Use a bed cradle to keep the bed clothes off the catheter.

Connect the catheter to the main fluid container and run in 1 litre quickly (in about 10 minutes). Warn the patient against sudden movements such as sitting up in bed. Allow the fluid to remain for a dwell time of 20 to 40 minutes and then drain it off into a sterile bag by gravity. A non-return valve in the bag lessens the risk of retrograde infection. Slight initial blood staining of the fluid is unimportant. Always leave a few ml of PD fluid in the drainage bag to serve as an airlock. Normally 1 or 2 litres of fluid should be cycled hourly depending on the metabolic needs. The aim should be to keep the plasma urea below 30 mmol/litre and the creatinine below 880 μmol-/litre.

The dialysate should be cultured every 24 hours and the tip of the catheter after removal. Every time any part of the circuit is opened spray the connection with Betadine. Disconnections are fewer if a 10 litre container (Difusor, Boots) is used with smaller bag between it and the patient. The Trocath can normally be kept in place for two to three weeks, *i.e.* during the whole of an episode of acute renal failure. For long-term dialysis a Silastic catheter is to be preferred (Heal, M. R., England, A. G. & Goldsmith, H. J. 1973, 'Four years' experience with indwelling Silastic cannulae for long-term peritoneal dialysis.' *British Medical Journal*, iv, 596-600.)

Difficulties
These are rarely encountered. If insertion proves too difficult try a site in the iliac fossa. It sometimes helps full insertion to have fluid running whilst introducing the catheter. A viscus may be perforated. Should this be the bladder your patient will be gratified by a sudden 2 litre 'diuresis'. Reinsert the Trocath elsewhere and put an indwelling catheter in the bladder. If faecal material is obtained ask a surgeon to come but leave the catheter *in situ* as it may help him to find the perforation. If he decides against operation remove the Trocath and insert a fresh one elsewhere adding gentamicin 6 mg per litre to the fluid. The commonest difficulty is failure to obtain an adequate outflow because of kinking, clinging omentum, fibrin clots or an airlock. If this happens withdraw the catheter a little but do not push it lest you introduce infection. If outflow remains poor or if the fluid contains much blood try forcible syringing with isosmotic sodium chloride solution. Large patients may need a large input before good drainage is established. Reinsertion in a second place may cause leakage into the abdominal wall from the first attempt. Discontinuance of PD for 24 hours will allow the first puncture to heal. If high dextrose fluid is used the blood sugar must be estimated daily and insulin given if need be to keep it below 14 mmol/litre. Too hypertonic a solution may cause pain and then 10 ml of 1 g/dl lignocaine may be added to 2 litres of infused fluid. During dialysis the sodium and fluid

balance needs careful watching. To treat uncontrollable hypertension use 1 litre of pure 5 g/dl dextrose to 4 litres of 130 mmol sodium dialysis fluid. To treat fluid retention or pulmonary oedema a mixture of high and low dextrose fluid in the proportion of 1:3 to 1:4 should be used with short dwell times.

PROCTOSCOPY

If a preliminary digital examination reveals a mass of faeces in the rectum empty it by enema or suppository or postpone the proctoscopy.

A full abdominal examination should include proctoscopy. As only the anal canal and rectal ampulla can be seen illumination can be from a lamp behind the doctor's head but some instruments have a built-in source of light. Let the patient be on his left side with his knees drawn up. With the obturator in position insert the lubricated instrument into the anus. As the sphincter relaxes tilt the instrument posteriorily and advance it till its flange is flush with the skin. Take out the obturator and note any pus, blood or mucus on its tip. Withdraw the proctoscope gently and slowly. The rectal mucosa is easily seen. Repeat the insertion but tell the patient to strain down during its withdrawal. This will enable you to see any internal haemorrhoids. (Sigmoidoscopy is a more expert procedure and is best done in the theatre by a surgeon experienced in it as it involves distention with air and possibly removal of tissue for biopsy.)

PLEURAL EXPLORATION, ASPIRATION AND BIOPSY

The first object is to find the nature of, rather than to show the presence of, pleural fluid. You should be fairly sure from clinical signs (cardiac displacement, stony dullness, silence on auscultation) that fluid is present before a needle is put in. X-ray confirmation is desirable. If pleural biopsy is desired the Abrams' needle can be used for aspiration as well but it is too large for routine aspiration only.

Pleural exploration

Put a pillow on a bed table and let the patient sit up and rest his arms on it. He may need support also. Most patients do not need premedication. The usual site for puncture is in the eighth or ninth space between the scapular and posterior axillary lines. Try to choose a place where dullness is marked and where there is a characteristic 'feel' in the intercostal space, but don't go too low or you will pierce the diaphragm. Prepare the skin (see p 82). Raise a wheal with 2 g/dl lignocaine and then infiltrate down to the pleura. Try to avoid the lower edge of the upper rib where the intercostal vessels are. Use a large needle attached by a three-way tap to a 20 ml syringe to penetrate the pleura and always make sure it is not blocked before use. Withdraw fluid and put some in a plain tube (for culture) and some in a citrate tube (for cytological examination). Seal the puncture site with a sprayed-on dressing (Nobecutane). If you fail try again one space higher.

If a bronchopleural fistula is suspected inject 5 to 10 ml of methylene blue into the pus. Blue sputum subsequently indicates a fistula.

Pleural aspiration

This is done in the same way as pleural exploration but a 50 ml syringe and two-way tap are used. Be prepared to spend considerable time in taking off the fluid but desist when coughing is troublesome or faintness comes on. (If the latter seems serious treat as for air embolism—see p 277.)

Replacement of fluid by air will often allow aspiration to go on longer than would be possible otherwise because the lung is prevented from expanding too quickly. A few syringesful of air (but fewer in number than the syringesful of liquid removed) are injected with the aspirating syringe. If a large amount of air is replaced it is well to put a second needle into the air pocket and connect to a pneumothorax apparatus. The amount of air should be adjusted so as to leave the pressure slightly negative. If there is any chance of a bronchopleural fistula always X-ray the chest before needling. You can then be certain that any gas in the pleura was not artificially introduced.

Pleural biopsy

It is common though not routine practice to take material for pleural biopsy with an Abrams' needle whenever a pleural effusion is tapped. Prepare the skin (see p 82) over a lower intercostal space posteriorly and infiltrate the tissues down to the pleura with 2 g/dl lignocaine. A small skin incision is made. The needle is introduced in the usual way and connected to a two-way tap for removal of some fluid. (There must be fluid between the lung and chest wall so as to avoid damage to the lung.) The inner component of the needle is drawn back so as to open the slot on the side of the needle and allow fluid to be removed. The needle is then withdrawn with the notch facing downwards (there is a small knob to indicate its position) so that this catches on the lower border of an intercostal space (upper border of rib below). The inner sharp-edged cannula is pushed home. It slices off a small (2 x 2 mm) piece of tissue held in the notch. The incision is closed by a fine suture. If the method is used in the absence of a pleural effusion a small pneumothorax has to be induced first.

PERICARDIAL PUNCTURE

When you do this for the first time it should always be under supervision. As circulatory failure may occur it is well to insert a board in the bed in case cardiac 'massage' is needed.

The sub-xiphoid route is preferred now that the risk of puncturing the heart is avoided by having an e.c.g. lead on the needle. This will show a strongly positive QRS deflection if the heart is touched. (The e.c.g. machine must be properly grounded, otherwise ventricular fibrillation could be induced).

An alternative route is via the fourth or fifth space just outside the apex beat or 2 cm to the left of the sternal edge (to avoid mammary vessels). The patient should lie down if possible so that the heart lies posteriorily. Shave and prepare the skin (see p 82). Infiltrate the site with 2 g/l lignocaine. This should not contain any adrenaline in case some might enter the heart. Use a 22 gauge lumbar puncture needle attached by a clip to a precordial e.c.g. lead. Enter the needle close to the upper border of a rib to avoid the vessels in the upper rib's groove. Should the fluid be too thick to aspirate the needle can be replaced by a larger one.

OBTAINING BLOOD FROM INFANTS

From the jugular veins

You should wait for a demonstration before attempting this yourself (though you could take blood from the umbilical vein in the cord at birth). You cannot expect to see or feel suitable veins under the age of 3 years and so you must use the internal jugular vein. Wrap the infant tightly in a blanket with arms inside. Put him on his back with his head just over the end of the couch. Turn his head to the opposite side to put the sternomastoid on the stretch. Insert the needle at its posterior border half way between the mastoid process and the sternal notch. While applying suction push the needle inwards keeping it closely on the underside of the muscle. (This is easy to feel with the needle point.) Blood will enter the syringe easily.

Sometimes the external jugular vein will stand out temptingly if compressed just above the clavicle. It slips away easily but if the skin is tensed it is possible to enter it. The needle should be inserted towards the chest but if more convenient it does not matter if you point it the other way.

From the heel

When not more than 1 ml of blood is needed and sterility is not important a heel prick may be used. Warm the foot by immersing it in hot water for two minutes. Rub it with spirit and quickly dry it. Smear the heel with petroleum jelly to facilitate the formation of discrete drops of blood. Milk the blood down the leg and grasp the heel between your thumb and index finger. Jab the heel sharply with a triangular needle or Autolet (Owen Mumford Ltd). Collect blood with a heparinised capillary tube or drop by drop directly into a bijou bottle.

ARTERIAL PUNCTURE

Palpate the brachial artery of the non-dominant arm and raise a wheal over it with 2 g/dl lignocaine (the radial artery of the wrist may also be used). Infiltrate the tissues down to the artery. Use heparin solution 500 units per ml to coat the inside of an all-glass well siliconed 10 ml syringe leaving sufficient to fill the dead space of the nozzle and needle. Introduce the needle (21 gauge) at an angle of 45 degrees and approach the artery keeping the left index finger just above the place where it is to be punctured. When the needle touches the artery pulsations are transmitted to it and when the lumen is entered blood rises easily into the syringe under its own pressure. Avoid suction for this would introduce bubbles of air. Remove 8 to 10 ml of blood taking a minute or more to do it. The patient should be breathing naturally. The operator or nurse should press on the artery afterwards for five minutes. Detach the needle and block the syringe with a match stick or specially blocked needle butt. Analysis should be made as soon as possible. If it has to be delayed the blood may be put into a bijou bottle so as to fill it. After centrifuging the plasma is drawn off and placed in the refrigerator. The inspired oxygen concentration should be included on the request form.

CAROTID SINUS MASSAGE

When properly applied this is a very effective method of vagal stimulation in patients with long narrow necks. It often fails because *pressure* only rather than *massage* is used. Give a sedative. The patient should lie flat (but when testing for hypersensitivity of the sinus he may stand). The head should be extended by a pillow under the neck and turned to one side. Face the patient and place the fingers of the left hand behind the neck and the thumb over the carotid sinus just below the angle of the jaw. The sinus may be felt as a bulge on the artery. Make firm strokes with the thumb up and down the artery for 3 or 4 cm while the patient counts aloud. Listen with a stethoscope all the time letting the patient hold the bell over his apex. Massage for five seconds in the first instance. If ineffective try the other side but never massage both sides together. Some operators prefer to place the fingers in front and the thumb behind. As fatal ventricular fibrillation has occasionally resulted e.c.g. monitoring is desirable so that stimulation can be stopped promptly if ventricular premature beats (especially 'R on T' extrasystoles) occur. In all cases facilities for cardiac resuscitation should be at hand.

BLOOD CULTURE (see also p 152)

Try to take blood at a time when the temperature is rising or at the onset of a rigor. Prepare the forearm skin thoroughly with soap and water and then as on p 82. Using a dry sterile syringe take 20 ml of blood from a vein. Inject 5 ml of blood through the rubber bung of both a bottle of glucose broth (for aerobes) and one containing heart-brain broth under negative pressure (for anaerobes). Label the bottles and return them to the incubator without delay. Always tell the pathologist what antibiotics have been given. When certain infections are suspected special media are used. Close liason with the microbiology department is desirable.

SWABS

A swab is made from non-absorbent cotton wool wrapped tightly round the end of a wire or wooden applicator and kept in a glass tube. Some microbiologists prefer swabs which have been dipped in serum and dried. Before swabbing dry areas moisten the swab with sterile water or broth. Consult the microbiologist first. He may prefer to take the swabs himself since results depend on the accuracy of swabbing and the speed of action in the laboratory. For virus infections a special transport medium must be used.

Throat swabs

Use a tongue depressor and a hand torch and let someone hold the patient's head. Swab a visible lesion if there is one. Otherwise start on the right tonsil, follow the arch to the left tonsil and end if possible by swabbing the posterior pharyngeal wall.

Nasopharyngeal swabs

These are used for meningococci, streptococci and Bordetella pertussis. In the oral route the tongue is depressed and the swab (on a long wire angled at the end) is passed behind the uvula. In infants a pernasal swab is best and is passed along the floor of the nose. It should be taken immediately after a paroxysm and the laboratory should be warned to pour a pertussis plate in readiness. In streptococcal carriers swab the nares as well and in staphylococcal carriers include the groins and perineum also.

Nasal swabs
Rub the swab on the wall of the vestibule (for staphylococci) and the turbinate bone (for nasal infections).

Laryngeal swabs
Wear a mask. Bend the wire holding the swabs. Grasp the tongue with a piece of gauze. Dip the swab in sterile water (sputum adheres best to a moist surface). Pass the swab down into the larynx and after the patient has coughed, withdraw and straighten it to allow insertion into its glass tube. It is usual to take two swabs. (These swabs have replaced the stomach washings test.)

Perianal swabs (for threadworm eggs)
Before the child has a bath or bowel action a cellophane swab is pressed against the skin of the anal margin. When the cellophane is removed and laid (skin side downwards) on a slide with a drop of 0.1 mol/l NaOH, any adherent eggs will be seen.

Vaginal and cervical swabs
Vaginal swabs are taken in the left lateral position and cervical swabs and scrapings in the lithotomy position. For cytology they should be taken in midcycle and before any manual examination is made. Use a speculum either dry or moistened with tepid water. The technique of using an Ayre's spatula should be learned from a colleague. The scraping should be firm and gentle with two complete rotations round the squamocolumnar junction of the cervix. For fixing instructions *see* *p* 138. Some operators use a dry brush on the cervix to obtain more cells which are added to the material on the slide.

For microbiology send one swab in special transport medium and use a second swab to make a film. In vaginal trichomoniasis it is best to take some vaginal discharge with a Pasteur pipette and, if necessary, injecting a little saline.

Skin and eye swabs
No special technique is required and the taking of these swabs is often done by the nursing staff. Unless discharge is profuse, however, swabs are likely to prove unsatisfactory. It is often better to send the patient to the laboratory to have material taken directly on a loop.

Rectal swabs

Ask the pathologist whether a swab will be enough. If it will not send some faeces. A specimen passed on to toilet paper in the lavatory pan and lifted out with a spatula is satisfactory.

RYLE'S TUBE

The nurses generally pass this but may call for your help. Don't take over immediately if there is obvious gagging and fighting against the tube. Allow a cooling off period and give a sedative i.m. (*see p* 81). Then respray the pharynx (including the nose if need be) with 4 g/dl lignocaine or let the patient suck an amethocaine lozenge. Pass the tube, lubricated with K-Y jelly, along the floor of the nose into the pharynx and give sips of water to help it go down. If these are contraindicated try a little persuasive pressure on the tube while the patient concentrates on taking deep breaths. It sometimes helps to give a lump of jelly to swallow with the tube. As the jelly cannot be distinguished from the tube this is more easily swallowed. The tube is marked with black rings: single at 35 cm, double at 50 cm and treble at 60 cm from the tip. Nostril to cardia is 45 cm. When the treble ring is 2 or 3 cm outside the nostril the tip is at the best depth for aspiration and the tube should be fixed to the face by strapping.

In the rare event of the tube being completely swallowed do not create an emergency by bringing the surgeon too soon. He can wait a long time (two weeks) if there are no ill effects. But you must take an X-ray film just before operation in case the tube has passed on.

PREPARATION FOR GASTROSCOPY

Explain the procedure to the patient and stress the fact that it is an examination and not an operation. See that the barium meal films are available. For a morning gastroscopy the patient must not take any food or drink after supper. If the examination is done in the afternoon a liquid breakfast is allowed. Your chief will tell you what premedication he prefers. This may be diazepam (Valium) 10 mg and atropine 0.5 mg i.m. half an hour before examination or i.v. (*see p* 81). Local anaesthesia is rarely needed but an amethocaine lozenge may be sucked or throat may be sprayed with a little 4 g/dl lignocaine. Gastric retention calls for the use of Señorans's evacuator or large syringe and possibly gastric lavage. No special measures are needed after examination beyond avoidance of hot drinks for a while if a local anaesthetic has been used.

ASPIRATION AND INJECTION OF JOINTS

Even though you do not work in a department of rheumatology it may fall to you to have to put a needle into a joint. As this can be very painful it is best to sedate an anxious patient (*see p* 81). The skin at the site of needling should be carefully prepared (*see p* 82). Wear a mask. Look up the landmarks in a book and palpate them on yourself or someone else first.

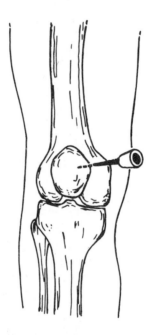

Fig. 3 The right knee extended. Anteromedial approach.

The knee

With the joint relaxed and slightly flexed enter the needle 1 or 2 cm from the medial border of the patella and direct it outwards and backwards between the patella and medial femoral condyle (Fig. 3). It is not quite so easy from the lateral side. If osteophytes make this injection difficult then the knee should be flexed to 90 degrees and the needle inserted through the outer or inner part of the tendon below the patella and directed backwards and slightly upwards (Fig. 4). An alternative site for obtaining fluid (and synovium for biopsy) is the suprapatellar pouch. The needle is directed through the quadriceps muscle on either side of its insertion into the patella. Other bursae round the knee may call for injection. The semimembranosus bursa is not normally continuous with the joint cavity and presents as a swelling in the popliteal fossa. After its careful palpation on the posteromedial aspect of the knee joint a needle may be directed into it. Needling through the popliteal space should be avoided and is not needed for bursae which are continuous with the joint.

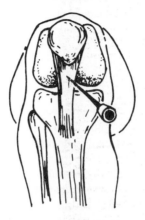

Fig. 4 The right knee flexed. Infrapatellar, anteromedial approach.

The elbow
Let the patient sit with his·elbow resting on a table and flexed to 90 degrees. Find the gap between the lower end of the lateral humeral

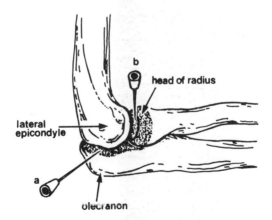

Fig. 5 The right elbow flexed. The stippled area shows the synovial membrane.

(Figs. 3, 4, 5 are from Cawley, M.I.D., 1974, in *British Journal of Hospital Medicine*, **2**, 744, by courtesy of the author and editor.)

condyle and the olecranon (Fig. 5). Insert the same needle as for the knee here and direct it anteromedially into the joint. Inject the steroid when the humeroulnar joint space is entered. The humeroradial and superior radioulnar joint spaces are continuous with that of the humeroulnar joint. If it is preferred to enter them separately the head of the radius is easy to feel and the joint is easily entered. When the olecranon bursa is involved it can be entered by a direct approach. For help with other joints you are referred to an article on 'Arthrocentesis', *British Journal of Hospital Medicine* by M.I.D. Cawley (1974), 2, 244.

NEEDLE BIOPSIES

These are outside your province until you have learned the technique from the registrar. But the preparation of the patient and supervision of the instrument tray can properly be regarded as your job. The type of needle used depends on the operator's preference. The Turner-Warwick apparatus can be used for most soft tissue biopsies. It is a special syringe with sharp trephine needles of various sizes. Suction is only used to retain the specimen within the needle so that the specimen is undistorted.

Bone marrow biopsy

Although it looks easy, aspiration of bone marrow is a very expert procedure if material of real value and not just blood is to be obtained. It is usually done by the haematologist. If it falls to your lot to provide a specimen you should certainly seek expert tuition first, particularly on how to make a film rapidly before the specimen is spoilt.

Liver biopsy

This is not a procedure to be undertaken lightly and you should only do it under supervision until you are expert yourself.

Preliminaries

The platelet count must be in the normal range for your laboratory. If the prothrombin time is not within 3 seconds of the control value a course of daily i.m. injections of phytomenadione (natural vitamin K_1 Konakion, Roche) should be given. Have the blood grouped and cross-matched. Remove any clinically obvious ascites by tapping or diuretics. Explain the procedure to the patient and give him a sedative (*see p* 81). Since breathing during the needling may tear the liver capsule make sure the patient can obey the commands to breathe in, breathe out and stop breathing. It may help if an assistant places the flat of his hand on the patient's chest to make sure that the breath is held.

The needle

For most cases a Tru-Cut needle (Travenol Laboratories) is best. It consists of a trocar and cannula with interlocking plastic mounts. The trocar has a 2 cm notch and slides within a cannula with a cutting edge. If there is cirrhosis some prefer to use a Vim-Silverman needle with twin blades which project beyond the end of an outer cannula. With a Menghini needle suction with a syringe must be maintained to get the specimen.

The needling

The patient must lie flat with his right side close to the edge of the bed. Tell him to put his right hand behind his head and turn his face to the left. Prepare the skin (*see p* 82). The usual puncture site is in the eighth or ninth space in the midaxillary line. Beware of going too far forwards as the gall bladder may be injured. Anaesthetise the tissues with 2 g/dl lignocaine using 10 to 20 ml in all (*see p* 119). Make a nick with a scalpel. Let the needle pass close to the upper border of the rib to avoid vessels in the intercostal groove above. If the subcostal route is chosen the liver must be easily palpable. If increased liver dullness is doubtful X-ray the abdomen to make sure there is no bowel between the ribs and the liver. Push the needle down to the pleura or liver surface. After a few practice breaths tell the patient, after breathing out, to stop breathing and then quickly advance the needle 3 or 4 cm into the liver. The depth can be limited by the index finger. Advance the Tru-Cut trocar fully and then the cannula to slice off the tissue in the notch and retain it. It is possible to obtain a further specimen by withdrawing the cannula and advancing the trocar again.

With suction techniques it is a disadvantage to withdraw material into the syringe and to obviate this some needles have a 'nail' to insert in the proximal end which stops the passage of solid matter but does not interfere with suction. If you should aspirate bile and have the presence of mind not to withdraw the needle, a little air may be injected since an X-ray film may then show up any gall stones.

With the Vim-Silverman needle the blades are pushed fully home into the liver and the cannula advanced to trap tissue between them. The needle is then twisted through 90 degrees and withdrawn. Specimens are put in fixative provided by the laboratory. Sometimes a small cage is provided to prevent them from breaking up.

After the puncture the patient should stay in hospital overnight and his pulse and blood pressure should be watched. The hazards are haemorrhage and biliary peritonitis but with careful selection and technique their incidence is low.

Lymph node biopsy

While you could probably remove a lymph node which is easily seen and felt or a piece of muscle these are operations best performed with your assistance by your surgical colleague under full operating theatre conditions. This is particularly so in the neck and axilla where a sound knowledge of anatomy is needed if mishaps are to be avoided. Premedication and a local anaesthetic with adrenaline is sufficient in most cases. Occasionally needle biopsy of a hard fixed gland is possible using a Turner-Warwick needle (p 102). In all cases the cosmetic result is important and thus skill in using fine atraumatic sutures is needed.

Muscle biopsy

Clinical examination by the dermatologist and sometimes electromy-ography will help to determine the site most likely to show the pathological lesions. A piece of overlying skin should be included. While it is often a surgical procedure there are special needling devices to do it. (For pleural biopsy see p 94 and peritoneal biopsy see p 89).

Skin biopsy

A small single lesion may be totally excised but in larger lesions an elliptical portion including some normal skin should be taken. Avoid the region of the sternum as incisions here are liable to keloid formation. Use 2 g/l lignocaine as a local anaesthetic but avoid adrenaline in lesions of the digits, nose, ears and genitalia. Excise a piece of tissue 1.0 by 0.5 cm. Go as deep as the subcutaneous fat and include some of it if panniculitis is suspected. Put the specimen into 10 per cent formalin in isosmotic sodium chloride solution. If an immu-nofluorescent technique is to be used e.g. for bullous lesions or collagen diseases ask the pathologist about the correct fixative. Dis-posable rotary punches are now available which will remove tissue up to 4 mm in diameter.

ELECTROENCEPHALOGRAPHY

Make an appointment in the department or at the hospital concerned and see that the patient presents himself at the appointed time having had no food or drink for the previous four hours. Anticonvulsive drugs should not be discontinued. The hair should be washed the night before but no grease applied.

ELECTROCARDIOGRAPHY TECHNIQUE

(This note is not concerned with the interpretation of the e.c.g. record. For help with this the HP is referred to one of the many books on the subject. *The ECG Made Easy* by J. R. Hampton, Churchill Livingstone, 1974 is recommended.)

You should follow the instructions provided by the maker of the machine you use. If it is the patient's first e.c.g. reassure him about it. Attach the electrodes to the hairless areas on the inner forearm just above the wrist and the outer aspects of the legs just above the ankle. Avoid bony points. Don't use solvents, except to remove liniments, and prepare the skin by a brisk dry rub with gauze. Rub in electrode jelly into the skin (preferably the non-sticky variety) with a spatula to decrease surface resistance but put it only on the area to which the electrode will be applied. The silver plus silver chloride electrodes should have been cleaned when last used. For chest leads suction electrodes are best. Disposable pre-gelled 'floating' electrodes are becoming popular. Localised shaving may be necessary. If an electrode cannot be kept in place it can be held through a swab or glove but not by the bare hand as this would spoil the record. Some electrodes can be held by an insulated handle. Jellied areas on the chest must not overlap or 'smudge' records may result which either resemble those of acute ischaemia or else show the same pattern in all the chest leads. If there is a tremor of the hand an electrode on the upper arm may yield a better record. You can attach an electrode to an amputation stump but if this is very short there is no objection to placing two electrodes on the opposite leg. Crossing of the leg leads does not matter but if the arm leads are reversed the record in lead I will be inverted.

In all modern e.c.g. machines the electric current generated by the heart beat is amplified several thousand times so that it can move a galvanometer coil whose electrically heated stylus writes on a moving strip of paper. An upward stroke represents a positive deflection. You may wonder why the lines on the record vary in thickness. This is because when ordinates represent differences in potential and abscissae represent time the greater the vertical displacement in a given distance the thinner will be the line.

The alloy electrodes are strapped to the right arm, left arm and left leg. Their wires have different colours (red for right arm and so on, but there is no universally agreed code). The electrodes are sometimes labelled as well. The screw attaching them to the wire must be tight. The electrode from the right leg is only to ground the patient and has no bearing on the record. The standard leads, I, II and III express the difference in potential between two electrodes:

Left arm (L) and right arm (R) is lead I
Left leg (F) and right arm (R) is lead II
Left leg (F) and left arm (L) is lead III

It was found by Wilson that when R, L and F were connected together the potential was close to zero and so this combination can function as an indifferent electrode completing the circuit but not affecting the record. The other (exploring) electrode is referred to as the voltage (V) lead and when taken from the right arm, left arm and left leg the record is referred to as VR, VL and VF. When the exploring electrode is on the chest it makes records for the positions V1 to V6.

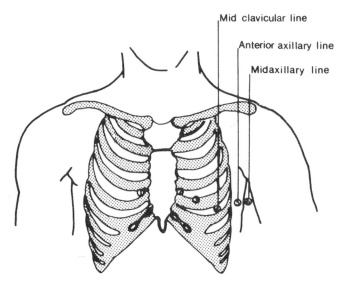

Mid clavicular line

Anterior axillary line

Midaxillary line

Fig. 6 The positions of the conventional chest leads. Note that the first intercostal space is immediately above and the second immediately below the sternal angle.

Unipolar limb leads were of inconveniently low voltage until Goldberger showed that when the connections between the limb to be used and the central terminal was broken the deflections were increased in size and these 'augmented' unipolar limb leads were referred to as a V leads thus: aVR, aVL and aVF. For routine purposes you should record from the following 12 leads: I, II, III, aVR, aVL, aVF, and the six chest leads from V1 to V6.

The chest leads are attached as shown in Fig. 6, *i.e.*

V1   Fourth intercostal space to the right of the sternum
V2   Fourth intercostal space to the left of the sternum
V3   Midway between V2 and V4
V4   Fifth intercostal space in midclavicular line
V5   Anterior axillary line level with V4 and V6
V6   Midaxillary line level with V5.

Make sure that the lead to the patient does not run parallel to a mains lead, as for example to a ripple bed. The patient must preferably be lying down unsupported by any muscular effort and relaxed. He must be warm and should keep still and silent during the recording. The leads are set by a selector switch. You must develop a technique by which you do not record until the switch has been turned to the appropriate lead. If you forget to do this and leave the switch at aVF for example, you may find you have identical records from V1 to V6. After moving the switch wait a few seconds for the stylus to return to the base line. A few centimetres of record is sufficient in most cases but a longer run may be needed in some arrhythmias. Wrong connections are a common source of error. If the chest electrodes are placed too high then the T waves will be inverted. The precordial electrode must be below the breast. In serial recordings exactly the same technique must be used each time to ensure comparable records. Before making a recording the instrument must be standardised so that 1 millivolt (mV) causes a deflection of 10 mm. In modern machines the sensitivity is pre-set and rarely needs altering. Dry multipoint electrodes have not proved a success and if you lack the jelly you can even use toothpaste.

BLOOD PRESSURE

In normal and hypertensive patients arterial blood pressure varies throughout the day being lowest at 0300 and highest at 1000 hours.

It is a good plan to measure the blood pressure early in the examination so that if it is high there will be time to do it again after the patient has settled down. Blood pressure, particularly the systolic, rises considerably with physical exercise and a little with mental effort and so the patient should have been semirecumbent for a short time and preferably have ceased smoking for an hour or so. If postural hypotension is suspected take readings in the standing and lying positions.

A mercury manometer is preferred. The cuff bladder length should be at least two-thirds the circumference of the arm and its width two-thirds the diameter of the arm to secure even occlusion. Too small a cuff may yield falsely high readings. (For a very obese arm the cuff may be placed round the forearm and the stethoscope over the radial artery.) Place the leads at the back of the upper arm so that they do not interfere with the stethoscope and secure the cuff with its Velcro or other fastening. Let the arm rest at heart level. Make a preliminary assessment of the systolic pressure by palpation of the radial artery. Then listen in the antecubital fossa where the brachial artery is easily palpable, inflating the cuff to 30 mmHg above this and listening as you reduce the pressure. The systolic pressure is that at which sounds reappear. Continue deflation. The diastolic pressure is that at which the sounds become muffled. Complete disappearance of the sounds should not be the criterion unless the phase of muffling cannot be detected. It is not unusual, even when there are no local abnormalities, for variation in the technique of cuff application to show differences between left and right. Fat arms often yield falsely high readings ('cuff hypertension'). It is well to record whether the patient was sitting or lying and which arm was used. The right brachial artery pressure is often higher than on the left, possibly because the innominate artery is more directly in line with the output of the left ventricle than is the left subclavian artery. A trick to intensify the end point is to ask the patient to hold his arm above his head and open and close his fist a dozen times and then relax before inflation in this position. Then lower the arm and proceed as before.

If and when the SI unit of pressure, the pascal (Pa), is adopted for blood pressure this will be expressed in kilopascals (kPa). One kPa is equivalent to 7.52 mm Hg.

RESPIRATORY FUNCTION TESTS

You should take the opportunity of making yourself familiar with the use of the recording spirometer, the Wright peak flow meter and the taking of arterial blood specimens for estimation of blood gases (*pp* 96 *and* 109). In case your laboratory does not measure blood gases the rebreathing method of estimating $PaCO_2$ should also be learned as it can be done anywhere with simple portable apparatus.

The forced expiratory time

Place a stethoscope over the trachea and using a stopwatch time a forced expiration. If this lasts more than 5 seconds there is significant airways obstruction, the degree of which is proportional to the duration of expiratory sounds.

Tests of ventilation

1. *Vital capacity (VC)*
    This is read from the expiratory spirogram produced by a recording

spirometer such as the Vitalograph. It is the volume of maximal unhurried expiration after a maximal inspiration. Normally it is about 6 litres for men and 4.5 for women but tables giving the figures for different heights and weights should be consulted. It is reduced in conditions which restrict the expansion of the lungs. (A few dummy runs should be made first.)

2. Forced vital capacity (FVC)

This also is measured by the recording spirometer and is the volume of air expelled by a forcible rapid expiration after a maximal inspiration. It is normally slightly less than the VC.

3. Forced expiration volume in 1 second (FEV₁)

This is read from the expiratory spirogram. It is the volume of air expired in the first second of the forced vital capacity test and so is a measure of flow rate. The normal FEV_1 is 5 litres in men and 4 litres in women but it varies with age and height. It is normally 75 per cent of the FVC and less in obstructive airways disease. The FEV_1 to FVC ratio is helpful, being low in obstructive lung disease and normal or high in chest restriction.

4. Peak expiratory flow rate (PEFR)

This also is a measure of airways obstruction. It is the maximum flow rate during forced expiration and is easily measured directly by the Wright peak flow meter or the smaller peak flow gauge, both of which are small and portable. Measuring the PEFR is more satisfactory than trying to derive it from the expiratory spirogram.

The Calculair electronic spirometer (Sandoz) gives many of the required measurements very quickly.

Blood gas analysis

This involves the taking of arterial blood (p 96) for PaO_2 $PaCO_2$) and pH.

Normal values:

1. Arterial oxygen saturation is normally 93 to 98 per cent at sea level.

2. Arterial oxygen tension PaO_2 is normally 10.6 to 13.2 kPa reducing to 9.97 to 11.97 kPa about age 60 and varying considerably with alveolar ventilation. The pH of arterial blood is usually estimated at the same time. Oxygen saturation is easier to measure than oxygen tension and often provides equally useful information. Its clinical estimation by cyanosis is rarely satisfactory.

3. Arterial CO_2 tension $PaCO_2$. Normally 4.5 to 6.1 kPa it is increased by hypoventilation and reduced by hyperventilation. Because of its high diffusibility it is not increased by disorders such as pulmonary fibrosis which impair gas transfer without reducing ventilation.

Transfer factor (Diffusing capacity for CO)
The single breath-holding method is most often used. The resting patient takes a deep breath of a gas mixture containing approximately 0.25 per cent CO. After 10 seconds breath-holding an alveolar sample is collected in a bag and having discarded the first 500 ml the CO content is determined by an infrared CO analyser. The normal diffusing capacity (dCO) is calculated from the difference between the CO content of the inspired gas and the alveolar sample. It varies with age, being 25 to 40 at age 20 and 18 to 30 at age 60. Impaired diffusing capacity is sometimes the chief physiological abormality and may be found when ventilatory tests are only moderately reduced.

LARYNGOTOMY AND TRACHEOSTOMY FOR ACUTE LARYNGEAL OBSTRUCTION

Desperately urgent relief of laryngeal obstruction is rarely needed (in 15 patients per million per annum) but you may be faced with it in a child who has inhaled an aniseed ball or when it complicates facial trauma in a road traffic accident. As there is no inspired air, relief cannot be obtained by coughing. The victim rapidly goes blue and unconscious. Within 4 minutes there will be irreparable brain damage. Upending the child may be tried but in most cases the cricothyroid membrane will have to be pierced. Identify the Adam's apple and the cricoid cartilage below it. Insert a large i.v. needle through the membrane between them angling it slightly downwards. If you direct it upwards you will damage the vocal cords. There will be a rush of air. Replace the needle by a plastic cannula and attach an Ambu bag via an adaptor. Having saved the patient's life by this 'mini-tracheostomy' ask your senior colleague to take over. Sometimes a special laryngotomy instrument with a knife and handled tracheostomy tube is available.

When obstruction threatens before becoming complete you can proceed less hurriedly. If you have to make a tracheostomy the following notes (studied beforehand) may help you.

With the patient lying flat put a pillow under his shoulders to extend the head. Tilt the feet downwards a little. An assistant must hold the head firmly in the midline. Local analgesia may be used if there is time.

An i.v. anaesthetic is dangerous and must not be used. On the other hand it is a help to give an inhalation non-explosive anaesthetic (halothane and oxygen). If right handed, stand on the patient's right and grasp the larynx with the left thumb and middle finger so that the index finger is on the cricoid. Make a skin incision vertically about 2.5 cm below the cricoid cartilage and incise the deeper tissues from the thyroid cartilage to the suprasternal notch. The wound fills with blood but ignore this. Bleeding will stop when the airway is clear. Deepen the incision until the rings of the trachea are felt. There is no need to divide the thyroid isthmus as the trachea can be suitably exposed below it. Incise the trachea through the second and third or third and fourth rings and twist the scalpel to make an opening. This controls the immediate emergency. Steps can now be taken to improve the operation and to make a good-sized hole in the trachea. Before the incision is lost the wound should be opened by using artery forceps and a tube pushed in. Opening through the first ring of the trachea should be avoided as it leads to stenosis. A stitch to fix the tube is wise. Gross bleeding should be controlled lest blood is aspirated.

OXYGEN ADMINISTRATION

You should be aware of the variables in oxygen administration and adopt a critical attitude to them. Oxygen can be given in high and low concentration and at atmospheric or increased pressure. Hyperbaric oxygen is used for repeated short periods but otherwise oxygen administration should be continuous and not intermittent. Adequate ventilation is very important and oxygen by itself is no substitute for it.

Oxygen in low concentration
Concentrations of 25 to 40 per cent are used for patients with hypoxaemia due to poor ventilation or uneven lung function, the aim being to prevent tissue hypoxia and hypercapnia while not removing the hypoxic drive.

Plastic tubes are satisfactory but even when the flow is 3 to 6 litres per minute a concentration in the inspired air of 30 to 60 per cent can only be achieved if the patient breathes through his nose. Humidification, preferably by an ultrasonic machine, is usual but is unnecessary with tubes and masks as it takes place in the nose. A single nasal tube should be placed so that its end is visible below the soft palate, but when both nostrils are used the tubes need not pass so far.

Various disposable masks deliver oxygen in the same concentration as tubes. The Venturi principle used in the Ventimask allows a jet of oxygen to entrain air from holes in the side of the mask at a fixed ratio of 1 in 10. The concentration of oxygen is constant because if its flow rate is increased to rates up to 8 litres per minute so is the amount of air entrained. A flow rate of 2 litres per minute is needed to deliver 24 per cent oxygen. To increase the concentration it is found best to use a range of masks delivering oxygen at fixed concentrations of 24, 28, 35 and 40 per cent. The flow of oxygen flushes away the expired CO_2. Be sure the mask used is the one you intend. In the Edinburgh mask air is breathed through a large hole in its front and oxygen is added by a jet. There is no reservoir. The concentration of oxygen inspired is varied by the flow rate but the concentration in the lungs varies inversely with ventilation. The Hudson multivent disposable mask allows a choice of oxygen concentration of 24 to 50 per cent. In the MC (Mary Catterall) small, close-fitting, leak-proof mask the effect of a valve is obtained by its shape and volume. A cone of inflowing oxygen is delivered direct to the nostrils and mouth. A small hole enables CO_2 to escape. A flow of 2 litres per minute gives a concentration of 35 per cent. For a patient who will not tolerate tubes or masks a simple measure is to enclose the head in folded X-ray films forming an inverted cone open at its base.

Oxygen tents are mainly of value for children and very disturbed patients. They do not provide higher concentrations of oxygen than simpler methods and there is a risk of accumulation of CO_2. The HAFOE (High Air Flow with Oxygen Enrichment) head and shoulders tent provides oxygen by the Venturi principle. Leakage is freely allowed and there is no need for cooling. The air flow is set at 8 litres per minute and the oxygen concentration regulated by varying the entrainment ratio.

Oxygen in high concentration
The main indications for this are CO poisoning and cardiac infarction. All masks delivering oxygen in high concentration use a high flow rate and store it in a bag during expiration from which it is inspired via a one-way valve. There is no rebreathing. Expiration is also via a one-way valve. In some masks the expiratory valve is replaced by a hole.

Hyperbaric oxygen
When this is indicated, as in CO poisoning, gas gangrene and acute vascular injuries, the patient is placed for two hours at a time in a special tank in which the pressure is built up. In the few hyperbaric rooms which exist it is the pressure of air which is built up. Since the pressure of oxygen does not improve ventilation hyperbaric apparatus is not used in respiratory failure. The hospital's office should know where the nearest hyperbaric centre is.

It should be scarcely necessary to add that to try to give oxygen by a tube and funnel held near the face is futile. A small rubber funnel with a flimsy edge and an expiratory hole may, however, be held closely over the face of an infant as a temporary measure.

Size of gas cylinders
Expressed in metric terms the normal capacity of cylinders is 682, 1365, 3410 and 6796 litres. Since oxygen does not liquefy at the pressure in cylinders (120 atmospheres), the volume of the contained gas is proportional to the pressure, and the pressure gauge is used to tell gas content. (This is not the case with gases like nitrous oxide which easily liquefy.)

Colours of gas cylinders
The house physician must be sure that any cylinder he uses contains the correct gas and there is a British Standard colour for each of them. Colour charts of gas cylinders are generally placed in anaesthetic rooms. The colours of gas cylinders used in medical wards are:

Oxygen. Black cylinder with white shoulder.

$O_2 + CO_2$. Black cylinder with grey and white shoulder quartering.

O_2+ *helium.* Black cylinder with brown and white shoulder quartering.

Air. Grey cylinder with black and white shoulder quartering.

Entonox (50 per cent N_2O in oxygen). Blue cylinder with blue and white shoulder quartering.

Warning
Oil and grease must not be used on oxygen taps and valves. Electrical apparatus of all kinds and anything liable to spark must be kept well away from the oxygen tent. Smoking and the use of matches and lighters must be absolutely forbidden near an oxygen tent or mask when in use. The house physician should satisfy himself that these points are clearly understood by all who use oxygen.

SUSPECTED SMALLPOX
You are unlikely ever to meet smallpox. Do not panic if you see a patient with chickenpox who has a vesicle on the palm and you think it is smallpox. Just sit down and think out quietly what may happen if it is smallpox. Do not move the patient or call your colleagues to have a look. They will not have seen a case either. Ring the Community Physician and let him decide what action is necessary.

NOTES ON INTRAVENOUS FEEDING
Complete or partial i.v. feeding is used by your surgical colleagues

after bowel resection and burns but it may be needed for gross undernutrition of medical origin and so some guidelines are given. You will probably use proprietary solutions but you should know the following basic facts about their constituents.

Glucose in 20 g/dl solution. Glucose provides 4 calories (16.8 joules) per g. The maximum amount utilisable is 0.5 g/kg/hour. If given too quickly the renal threshold will be exceeded and some will be lost. The rate of administration should be kept below 0.25g per kg per hour. (Fructose should only be considered if the patient is over 12 and not acidotic or with liver problems.) Insulin may be needed.

Fat emulsion. Fat provides 9 calories per g. Not more than 2g per kg body weight should be given in 24 hours. To ensure that it is fully utilised 30 per cent of the total calorie intake must be provided by carbohydrate. A blood sample must be taken before each infusion as it must not be repeated until any hyperlipaemia (milkiness) has cleared.

Amino acid solutions. The requirement is 1g per kg per day and for each gram given 200 calories must be provided.

Glucose and amino-acid solutions may be given together but fat emulsions must be given separately.

Ethyl alcohol (ethanol) is a source of calories in some proprietary solutions. It should only be given with amino-acids. One gram of ethanol provides 7 calories.

Basic requirements for an adult per kg body weight per day are:
Calories, 30
Fluid, 30 ml
Carbohydrate, 2.0 g
Fat, 2.0 g
Amino acids, 1.0 g

In addition vitamins (i.m.) and electrolytes (i.v.) will be needed. (The potassium requirement is 0.8 mmol/kg/day.)

Intravenous feeding does not cause acid-base disturbances but as all solutions are hyperosmolar compared with plasma there is a tendency to hyperosmolality.

Technique

The subclavian vein is used (*see p* 86). Strict asepsis must be observed. In some hospitals a doctor-nurse-technician team wearing gowns, masks and gloves is responsible for the procedure. The patient also should wear a mask. A Vicro Centrasil silicone elastomer catheter (Travenol) (radio-opaque) is generally used. There is also a longer Vygon silicone catheter (Code 181. 17 UK). When multiple drips are being used a Vygon 5-way connector (Code 873.04) close to the vein avoids interactions between mixing solutions before the vein is reached. Infusion of hypertonic solutions should never be started until the correct placement of the catheter has been checked radiologically. Any additions such as vitamins should be made in the pharmacy and never injected into the drip line. Skin cleansing should be as on *p* 82. The entry site should be covered with gauze and then sprayed with a bactericidal sealing solution. In some units measures to lessen the risk of infection are to put a micropore filter in the line and to tunnel the catheter subcutaneously from an entry point lower down on the chest wall.

CENTRAL VENOUS PRESSURE (C.V.P.)

When raised an estimate of the height of the C.V.P. can be obtained in a patient with head and shoulders raised to about 30 degrees, by measuring the horizontal height above the sternal angle of the upper end of the engorged part of the external jugular vein, and adding 2 cm. A curved graduated plastic tube whose ends are placed in these points enables raised C.V.P. to be estimated at the bedside. For more accurate measurement an i.v. catheter is necessary (*see p* 84).

Technique

Choose the basilic vein at the elbow or the right internal jugular vein in the neck. (Avoid the cephalic vein because of its valves and the kink at the deltopectoral groove.) Use a Medicut needle and insert a long tube through its cannula. The end of the C.V.P. tube should be at the junction of the superior vena cava and the right atrium. (If it is in the right atrium puncture of the wall is a possible complication). Fill the tube with sterile isosmotic sodium chloride solution. Prepare the skin (*see p* 82) and infiltrate with 2 g/dl lignocaine and isolate the vein through a 1 cm incision. Make a small opening in it with scissors and pass the tube till its end is judged to be at the lower border of the superior vena cava. Next demonstrate a free respiratory rise and fall of blood. To do this remove the cap at the end of the tube and let blood flow till it can be seen at the elbow. Ask the patient to take a few deep breaths and movement of the blood column will then be seen. If there is pulsation withdraw the tube a bit. Tie in the tube by proximal and distal ligatures of Dexon 3/0. Connect the tube to a Travenol Laboratories FKC0121, venous pressure manometer set. By use of the tap and flow-clip fill its tubes with fluid from the bottle. Make an indelible X mark on the patient's chest in the midaxillary line. This level is midway between the spine and the sternum and corresponds to the level of the right atrium. Put the self-adhesive centimetre scale on the upright of the drip stand and adjust it so that the 0 cm mark is opposite the X on the chest wall.

Turn the tap to connect the manometer line and read the C.V.P. in cm of saline. A rise and fall of 1 cm with respiration is easily seen. A little methylene blue in the manometer arm is a help. If the patient moves or sits up 0 cm must be levelled to X before reading the pressure. The position of the tube tip should be checked by X-rays. The apparatus should be tested by running in rapidly 100 ml of isosmotic sodium chloride solution. This should cause a rise of 3 cm in the C.V.P.

The C.V.P. measures the balance between the return of blood to the heart and the heart's capacity to expel it. While it is a valuable guide in hypovolaemic shock it is not the sole criterion of the necessity for fluid replacement. Normally a tube whose end is in the proximal superior vena cava shows a pressure of 6.2 ± 1.5 cm saline. At the sternal angle it is up to 3 cm. When the C.V.P. is low (-2 to 4 cm) it indicates the need for fluid replacement. When it is high (>15 cm) the patient is either in cardiac failure or is being overloaded. Airways obstruction and I.P.P.V. raise the C.V.P.

Difficulties

1. Irregular movement of the manometer column indicates myocardial irritation by the end of the tube. Adjust the position.

2. Overloading. This may occur if the manometer line is not working and gives a false low reading. You may also allow overloading to develop if you don't take pressure readings often enough.

SKIN TESTING

This may be by prick, intracutaneous injection or patch.

Prick test

This is used in the diagnosis of allergic conditions of the 'anaphylactic' type—hay fever, allergic rhinitis and allergic asthma. It may show a positive reaction in farmer's lung and aspergillosis. Make a list of the allergies for which it is proposed to test. Clean the volar surface of the forearm or the interscapular area with methylated spirit 70 per cent v/v and let it dry. Put a drop of saline followed by drops of the testing materials on the skin in a row 15mm apart in the order on the list. Make a prick with a sterile Hagedorn needle or disposable lancet through each drop. Hold the needle almost parallel to the skin. The prick should be minimal, practically painless and entirely bloodless. Wipe the needle thoroughly with a moist swab between each prick and use a new one for each patient. A positive reaction will appear within 20 minutes as an urticarial wheal clearly differing from the reaction to that of the control saline. A record may be made by outlining the wheals with a Biro pen, covering these with Sellotape and transferring the strip to the case sheet. In farmer's lung and aspergillosis a different type of allergic reaction is involved. It may take several hours to develop and is seen as a diffuse swelling.

Intracutaneous test

This should be used with caution and in most cases only when the prick test is negative. Severe reactions to tuberculin and to Casoni (hydatid), Kveim (sarcoidosis), Frei (lymphogranuloma venereum) and Toxocara antigens are unlikely. The solutions used are more dilute than those for the prick tests. A dose of 0.1 to 0.2 ml is injected into but not through the skin and should raise a small bleb. A positive reaction may occur rapidly and, with pollens, moulds and some dietary allergens, may cause generalised urticaria and even anaphylaxis. The tuberculin type of reaction occurs in 24 to 48 hours.

Patch test

This is used to diagnose a contact type of allergy ('contact dermatitis'). A small amount of the suspected offender (garment, leaf, plastic material or a liquid) is placed on the skin and covered with a square of gauze held in place with tape. It is left for 24 hours and then inspected by lifting the corner. If nothing shows it is left for another 24 to 48 hours. A positive result is a clearly marked area of erythema or eczema corresponding to the testing material. If undue irritation is felt before 24 hours have elapsed the patient should remove the patch and wash the area.

Dependable testing solutions are available commercially. They are expensive and deteriorate with age. It is therefore unnecessary to keep a large stock for routine work. A reasonable assembly for prick and patch tests is:

Control saline
Domestic: Feathers, Horsehair, Household mite.
Pets: Cat, dog, budgerigar, rabbit, hamster, guinea pig.
General: Grass pollen, tree pollen, *Aspergillus fumigatus,* farmer's lung moulds.
Dietetic: Milk, egg white, egg yolk, fish, nuts.
Patch tests: Paraphenylene diamine 2 per cent in Vaseline (hair

dyes) and nickel sulphate 5 g/dl aqueous solution (metal clips and costume jewelry).

Highly sensitive persons may react to a prick test with generalised urticaria. Treatment as described under serum administration (*p* 118) may be necessary. If claims for damages are contemplated as for example in 'bra dermatitis', assemble the evidence with anxious care and take colour photographs if possible.

SERUM ADMINISTRATION

Always test first for hypersensitivity. Puncture the forearm with a hypodermic needle (control) and do it again through a drop of serum. Redness and wheal formation in the test arm but not the control indicate sensitivity. If it is present or if your patient is subject to asthma or urticaria or gives a history of previous reactions to serum or drugs be very cautious about injecting foreign serum. The first dose should be 0.2 ml of a 1 in 10 dilution in isosmotic sodium chloride solution subcutaneously. If all goes well after 15 minutes you can inject 0.2 ml of a 1 in 5 dilution and lastly 0.1 ml of undiluted serum. Any reaction calls for abandonment or more graduated doses in slow sequence. When there is no reaction to 0.1 ml of undiluted serum you can go ahead and give the whole dose. For a severe anaphylactic reaction give 0.3 ml Adrenaline Injection BP (1 in 1 000) subcutaneously. Never be tempted to give it i. v. You may have to use the other drugs on the anaphylaxis tray.

Anaphylaxis tray
This should always be ready when serum is given. It should have on it: Adrenaline Injection BP (1 in 1 000), aminophylline 250 mg in 10 ml ampoules, hydrocortisone sodium succinate (Efcortelan soluble, Glaxo) 100 mg ampoules with 2 ml ampoules of water for injection, chlorpheniramine (Piriton) 10 mg ampoules for i.m. injections as well as the necessary syringes and needles, and an airway, tracheostomy instruments and a cutting down set. Oxygen and suction should be at hand. You may have to call the 'May Day' team.

TUBERCULIN TESTING

Intradermal (Mantoux)
A disposable syringe should be used but if it has to be a glass one it must not be used for any other purpose as it is very difficult to rid it of tuberculin. Use tuberculin PPD 1 in 1 000 (= 10 tuberculin units) supplied in 1 ml ampoules. Clean the skin of the flexor surface of the

forearm with 70 per cent v/v methylated spirit and let it dry. Inject 0.1 ml intradermally. Read the result at 72 hours. If positive there is an area of induration not less than 6 mm in diameter. Redness without oedema is not significant.

Multiple puncture (Heaf test)
Use a solution of PPD containing 2.0 mg per ml (100000 tuberculin units). This gives results equivalent to the intradermal test using 50 tuberculin units. Cleanse the skin of the forearm. Apply the PPD solution with a sterile loop or glass rod and spread it over an area of 1 cm². The gun should have been sterilised by immersing in methylated spirit and burning it off. Set it to puncture to a depth of 2 mm for patients over 2 years. Set it at 1 mm for patients under 2 years. Apply the head and release the needles. Let the skin dry. No dressing is needed. Read the results at 4 to 7 days. Induration which can be felt is an essential feature of a positive result. There should be four or more palpable papules which may coalesce.

LOCAL ANALGESIA

You should be aware of the maximum safe dose of any local analgesic you use, and its toxic effects. Always read the label yourself. Never dismiss lightly a patient's statement that he had a reaction to an injection previously. Give him a small dose (0.5 ml of a 1 g/dl solution) and wait. Never inject cocaine and always avoid it and adrenaline in any patient taking a monoamine oxidase inhibitor.

The dose of a local analgesic varies with a patient's weight, general condition, vascularity of tissues and with its admixture or not with adrenaline. Toxicity increases with concentration in geometrical and not in arithmetical progression and so a 2 g/dl solution is four times more toxic than a 1 g/dl solution. Always use added adrenaline except where contraindicated (by ischaemic heart disease, a peripheral part —toe, finger, penis— or the probable use of halothane or trichloroethylene).

Lignocaine
This is the most generally used local analgesic. The maximum safe dose for a 70 kg man is 500 mg with adrenaline (7 mg/kg) or 200 mg without adrenaline (3 mg/kg). The safe volume is inject is:

Concentration	Volume of solution (ml)
0.5 g/dl with adrenaline	100
1.0 g/dl with adrenaline	50

Concentration	Volume of solution (ml)
2.0 g/dl with adrenaline	25
0.5 g/dl without adrenaline	40
1.0 g/dl without adrenaline	20
2.0 g/dl without adrenaline	10

Other local analgesics
Maximum safe doses are:

Prilocaine (Citanest)—600 mg with adrenaline
  —400 mg without adrenaline
Procaine—200 ml of a 0.5 g/dl solution.
Amethocaine (for surface analgesia)—Not more than 80 mg

All doses apply to adults. Children and aged, shocked and hypothyroid patients are less tolerant. Patients with myasthenia gravis are specially liable to collapse. In nervous patients a preliminary dose of diazepam is wise (*see p* 81). If you have to add the adrenaline yourself four drops of 1 in 1000 solution from a 12 needle added to 25 ml of analgesic solution gives the usual strength of 1 in 250000. The maximum safe dose of adrenaline is 0.5 ml of 1 in 1000 solution.

Symptoms and treatment of overdosage
Early symptoms are itching, sneezing and wheezing. Talkativeness, sweating and restlessness warn of cerebral effects and may be followed by delirium and convulsions. Lower the head. Give oxygen. If twitchings and convulsions occur call the anaesthetist with a view to thiopentone or suxamethonium.

GROUPING AND CROSS MATCHING OF BLOOD

You should not attempt these procedures yourself but leave them to the pathologist or an experienced technician. Read the *Notes on Transfusion* (MRC publication 36) provided by the Department of Health. Do not unnecessarily hurry the laboratory to provide compatible blood. Try to order it a full day in advance of need. It may be your job to obtain the blood sample for cross matching. Send 10 ml in a plain bottle. Tell the pathologist about previous transfusions, pregnancies, miscarriages or injections of blood. Also warn him if the patient is taking methyldopa (Aldomet). If you are going to give Dextran take your sample first. If a newborn baby needs transfusion cross-matching must be done against the mother's and not the baby's blood because any antibody it contains will have arrived across the placenta.

You can be of great help by attending carefully to non-technical details. The greatest risk nowadays lies in the journey of blood from the refrigerator to the bedside. So study carefully the procedure used in your hospital. Make sure that the group shown on the blood bag label is the same as that of the recipient. Colour coding of blood bag labels is: AB, white; A yellow; B, pale red; O, blue. If blood is Rh negative the label has a vertical red bar.

Only a responsible person should collect blood from the bank. After ensuring that he has the right bag he should sign the register. Two responsible people should check at the bedside the name, group, expiry date and number of the bag and compare these data with the patient's notes. Both should then sign the label.

TRANSFUSION REACTIONS

Pyrexia
Some patients show a mild pyrexia during transfusion. If it is not above 38.3°C and there are no other symptoms transfusion can continue. But don't give more than a dose of aspirin lest drugs mask a serious reaction. Pyrexia which recurs with each transfusion should be investigated by the pathologist.

Allergic reactions
Urticaria and bronchial spasm only arise rarely and then in patients with a history of allergy. If a reaction is mild then slowing the transfusion and giving an antihistamine drug is sufficient. Don't add drugs to the blood in the bottle.

Incompatible transfusion reaction
This is a serious but avoidable accident. There is pyrexia (above 38.3°C), backache, headache, nausea and a feeling of constriction in the chest. Circulatory collapse and haemoglobinuria may follow. Stop the transfusion at once. Treat for circulatory collapse and warn the renal dialysis unit. Further measures will be decided on by your chief. you can help by providing evidence for the investigation which will follow. The pathologist will require:

1. A pre-transfusion specimen of the recipient's blood.
2. A sample from the donor bag.
3. A post-transfusion specimen of the recipient's blood in a citrate tube and a clotted (10 to 20 ml) specimen.
4. Any urine passed during and for 24 hours after transfusion.

Out-dated blood
This will cause haemoglobinuria and jaundice but without the symptoms of a true transfusion reaction.

Potassium poisoning
During storage potassium leaves red cells and enters the plasma where its level may rise to 20 mmol/litre after 20 days. Massive transfusion of such blood will raise the recipient's plasma potassium level. At 10 mmol/litre ventricular fibrillation and circulatory arrest may follow. If this threatens give 100 ml of dextrose 50 g/dl, 50 units of insulin and 20 ml of calcium gluconate (10g/dl) i.v. Failing this arrange for dialysis.

Warmed blood
Warming is unnecessary and unwise in most cases and should only be ordered by the consultant. Special methods are needed. Warmed unused blood must be discarded.

Haemolysis
This is shown by a reddish discolouration of normally straw-coloured plasma just above the cell layer. Such blood should not be used.

Bacterial contamination
This is an ever-present hazard. Some organisms will grow in blood if it is kept at room temperature for a time. Blood should not be out of the refrigerator for more than 30 minutes on any occasion. Bags which have been punctured and not used within 24 hours should not be saved for future use even though kept at 4°C. They should be returned to the Blood Transfusion Centre. Partly used bags must never be reused. Never put blood bags in the domestic-type refrigerator in the ward. This should be labelled 'Not for storage of blood for transfusion'.

Circulatory overloading
This results from too rapid transfusion of too much blood in a patient with a failing heart and causes cough, frothy sputum, dyspnoea and basal râles. The central venous pressure (p 115) rises. Stop the transfusion. Remove blood or apply tourniquets to the legs and give morphine and a diuretic oxygen.

Massive transfusion
Give 10 ml calcium gluconate 10 g/dl i.v. following the third litre (6 units) of whole blood to counteract the effect of added citrate. Since the levels of platelets and factors V and VIII decrease rapidly in stored

blood, bleeding disorders may result from massive blood transfusion. Do not transfuse blood with added citrate to patients with severe liver disease. Use heparinised blood instead.

LUMBAR PUNCTURE

Contraindications

Lumbar puncture should be avoided in the ward if there is any suspicion of papilloedema on ophthalmoscopy and even if the history is suggestive of raised intracranial pressure although there is not yet any swelling of the disc. Lumbar puncture in such cases should only be done where there are full neurosurgical facilities.

Preparation

The secret of success is to start with the patient in the correct position. As a needle coming from behind can be very worrying plentiful reassurance is wise. A very nervous patient should be sedated (*see p* 81).

Position of patient

If you are right-handed your patient should lie on his left side with his buttocks and shoulder on the hard edge of the bed. If the mattress sags

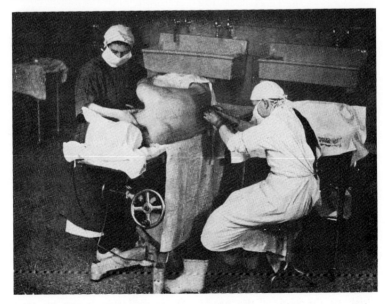

Fig. 7 Position for lumbar puncture. The operator's eyes are behind the hub of the needle so that he can look along the line of the shaft.
(Lumbar puncture and spinal analgesia. Macintosh and Lee.)

put fracture boards under it but it would be better to use an operating table (Fig. 7). The long axis of the spine should be horizontal and the plane of the iliac crests vertical. The spine must be fully but not forcibly flexed and the patient should be asked to get his chin as near to his knees as possible. Tell him to arch his back like a cat. A roller towel placed round the neck and knees and tightened by twisting with a rod sometimes helps to obtain and maintain the flexed position. A pillow between the legs will prevent the patient from rolling over. When landmarks are uncertain the sitting position can make the puncture easier.

Site of puncture

The usual site is the space between the spines of the third and fourth lumbar vertebrae. This space is on Tuffier's line passing through the highest points of both iliac crests. It crosses the spine just above the fourth lumbar vertebral spine. Figure 8 shows the correct position of the vertebrae. Never tap higher than the space between the second and third vertebrae or the cord will be damaged.

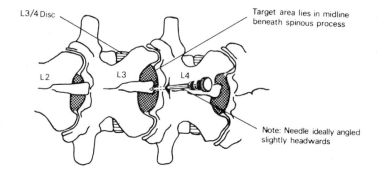

Fig. 8 Vertebral position with patient correctly placed. (Courtesy of *Teach-in* and Dr John Patten.)

The puncture

Sit on a stool so that you can look along the line of the needle. A stout, size 18 needle can be used if the spine is stiff and difficulty is expected. Otherwise a fine (20 gauge) needle is to be preferred such as the disposable Monoject (Sherwood Industries). The stilette must fit flush to the end of the needle. Make sure that it can be easily withdrawn. In case the needle bends it is a good plan to use a needle director or even a i.v. cannula. This is inserted down as far as the ligamentum flavum and the puncture is made by a fine needle passed down it.

Prepare the skin (*see p* 82). Everything should be dry including your hands. Gloves are not essential and instead of them a sterile gown may be used through which the needle is held and the skin palpated. Hold the skin taut between the thumb and the index so that the entry point does not move after raising a small wheal with 2 g/dl lignocaine over the junction of the lower and middle thirds of the interspace. Pierce the skin through the wheal by giving the needle a rolling motion. Then check that the direction of the needle is correct and push it through the interspinous ligament making sure that it is kept at right angles to the spine. Push on inclining the needle slightly towards the head and pierce the ligamentum flavum with a slight 'give'. (This is not always felt if the needle is very sharp.) You may have entered the subdural space already so pull out the stilette. Fluid may flow. If it does not, rotate the needle in case a nerve root is impinging on it. Always replace the stilette before advancing further by about 2 mm. Continue until fluid emerges. With a sharp needle there is danger of going too far and puncturing the veins in the ventral epidural space rather than not going far enough. A refinement to prevent overpenetration is to remove the stilette when the ligament is reached and to put a drop of saline in the butt of the needle. When the tip enters the extradural space the saline is drawn inwards by negative pressure. Take 5 ml of fluid into each of two specimen bottles and 2 ml into a fluoride bottle for glucose estimation. Withdraw the needle. There is no need to press on the site. Apply an adhesive dressing.

Difficulties

1. No fluid flows. Replace the stilette. Advance the needle a few millimetres and rotate it in case a nerve root is obstructing it. Never try aspiration by a syringe.

2. Bone is encountered. This usually means that flexion is incomplete. Withdraw the needle and adjust the position.

3. Blood appears. If it is only a few drops and then nothing more it means that the needle has not gone far enough but is in the subdural space.

'Bloody tap' (*see also p* 211)

If the fluid is bloodstained you must decide whether this is due to trauma or spontaneous subarachnoid haemorrhage. Traumatic bleeding often shows as a swirl and clears as the fluid drains. If in doubt take specimens into three numbered tubes and ask for red cell counts on them. A lightening colour and a diminishing count indicate traumatic blood. Clotting may occur if bleeding was due to trauma and then, if centrifuged, the supernatant fluid will be colourless. In subarachnoid haemorrhage clotting does not occur and the supernatant fluid becomes yellow (a simpler word than xanthochromic) after a few hours for a week or two. Red cells disappear in 5 to 10 days.

Pressure of c.s.f.
Ritual measurement of c.s.f. pressure and Queckenstedt's test are to be discouraged. It is sufficient to show the normal response of a brisk rise of 10 mm or so when a patient, breathing quietly, gives a cough.

Post-puncture headache
Measures to avoid this are:

1. Use as small bore a needle as possible.
2. Keep the bevel vertical so that by splitting the fibres of the ligamentum flavum rather than cutting across them the hole in the ligament is more likely to close.
3. Make the patient lie down, preferably prone, for 1 to 4 hours after puncture.

THE HOUSE PHYSICIAN AND THE X-RAY DEPARTMENT

Details of the preparation for various X-ray examinations are not given because they vary from hospital to hospital and are the concern of the radiologist. You should make yourself familiar with his preferences.

Request forms
Fill in the details with care. If you have two patients of the same name use whatever system exists in your hospital to alert the X-ray department to the fact. Give the date and place of X-ray examinations made before the current series. Say when the operation was done. (Gas under the diaphragm next day will not worry the radiologist as gas found a week later would.) In accident cases give the time of injury. Make a note about stilboestrol and cortisone as these can change the appearance of bones. Indicate how the patient will reach the department, *i.e.* stretcher, chair, walking or 'carry'.

Casualty
If the patient remains your responsibility after being X-rayed, *e.g.* a casualty case, always see the radiologist's report later in case you have overlooked, for example, a fracture. Be especially careful about wrists. A fracture of the scaphoid is the one most often missed.

Goggles
If you go to watch the patient being screened put on your dark goggles well beforehand unless an image intensifier is in use. It is wise to leave your camera behind.

Examining films
See that wet films are kept apart, for if they touch they will stick and be ruined. The first thing to do with a film is to make sure it refers to the patient in question. Be particularly watchful if there are two patients of the same name and if the clinical and X-ray findings are inexplicably at variance look at the film before a good bright viewing box. Only base a 'no fracture' opinion on a dry film.

Chest
No special preparation is needed. Postero-anterior films are taken in the department and are made in full inspiration to show as much of the lungs as possible. If a small pneumothorax is suspected it may only be apparent on a film taken in expiration. Do not ask for lateral views until the PA film has been seen. 'Portable' films are anteroposterior. Do not ask for them unless the patient really cannot go to the department. A feeble patient may need assistance from you or the nurse during his examination. In this event lead aprons should be worn.

Foreign bodies
If inhaled or 'swallowed' X-ray the chest at once. There is less urgency about a definitely swallowed foreign body but it is very important to be sure it is not in the lungs.

Skull
In at least 10 per cent of cases of head injury there is intracranial bleeding but no bone injury. To be of real help skull films must be carefully taken preferably when the patient is co-operative. So do not rush to X-ray the head after an injury merely on medicolegal grounds. If you can say that you omitted to X-ray the head for good reasons you have nothing to fear. Whether to request a brain scan is for your chief to decide.

Spine
In back injuries always see that the dorsal spine is X-rayed no matter where the pain is. A canvas trolley top with poles allows patients with suspected spinal injuries to be X-rayed with a minimum of risk.

Ribs

Fractured ribs may not be shown by X-rays until a few days after an injury. So the early diagnosis should be made on clinical grounds and you should be more concerned about the state of the lungs than about whether a rib is cracked or not.

Shoulders

Never X-ray a painful shoulder without X-raying the chest as well.

Abdomen

If you ask for a plain film of an 'acute abdomen' see that the chest is done also and in the erect position. (Gas under the diaphragm shows best on the chest film.) Sit the patient up for a few minutes first. It is well to ask for erect and supine films of the abdomen.

I.V.U. (Intravenous urogram)

In many hospitals it is the house physician's job to inject the contrast medium but you should do more than merely this. You should always know why the i.v.u. is being done and see the plain film in case it is unsatisfactory and has to be repeated. You should not proceed if the blood urea is over 15 mmol/l, as if you did the result would unsatisfactory. The dose of contrast medium should contain up to 600 mg iodine per kg body weight. Films are taken at 5, 10 and 45 minutes. The first one may be poor because a fall of blood pressure lowers the filtration rate. If it is very poor more contrast medium can be given. Very few patients even if there is an allergic history show any allergic reaction. Pre-testing and prophylactic antihistamines are unhelpful. Should more than transient nausea and flushing occur give hydrocortisone 100 mg i.v. When relevant ask for a post-micturition film to show any residual urine.

Barium meal

Always give details of what is suspected clinically. Don't ask routinely for a barium meal and follow through. If intestinal obstruction is a possibility consult the radiologist. There are contrast media which can be used without risk in suspected obstruction. If a cholecystogram is likely to be wanted also, do it before the barium meal to avoid delay in waiting for the barium to clear.

Barium enema

Sigmoidoscopy should be done before rather than after a barium enema.

Cholecystograms

The oral method is intended to show the gall bladder but is of no value in the jaundiced patient. It is best done two or three weeks after the attack of gall bladder trouble. The i.v. method is intended to show the bile ducts and again is best done two or three weeks after the disturbance which suggested it. The percutaneous transhepatic cholangiogram in patients with obstructive jaundice should only be made just prior to operation.

Radiological hazards in women

In all female patients of reproductive capacity, *i.e.* aged 12 to 50, the chance of irradiation of a pregnancy should be reduced. There is a chain of responsibility in achieving this. The woman should be told that some examinations may be harmful and the warning notice in the department should be in such terms as 'If you think or know you are pregnant you must warn the radiographer'. The requesting doctor should put the date of the last menstrual period on his request form. (This may have a space labelled LMP to remind him).

Any X-ray examination of the abdomen should be done within the 10 days following the first day of the LMP. If you chief decided that X-ray examination is needed irrespective of possible pregnancy he should mark the form, 'Ignore the 10 day rule'. You must use your common sense. No action is needed if the woman is menstruating at the time; has had a hysterectomy or sterilising operation; has used a contraceptive device or has been 'on the pill' successfully for three months or more, or denies recent sexual intercourse. But beware of patients who speak little English or who do not easily understand (*see pp* 2 & 11). Some hospitals, therefore, to narrow down the number of women to whom the rule applies, give the patient a form on which she states the first day of the last period and whether there is any possibility of pregnancy having occurred.

Computerised tomography

Neurological practice in particular has been greatly changed by this technique which is used to display tissues with differing X-ray absorption coefficients. No special preparation is required for examination of the brain or orbit. A laxative should be given two nights before a pelvic scan. No fresh fruit, vegetables, baked beans or fizzy drinks should be taken for two days before an abdominal scan (to reduce bowel gas). Contrast enhancement with Conray (brain examination) or Gastrografin (abdominal examination) and other measures are dealt with in the X-ray department.

Emergencies in the X-ray department
You may be involved in an emergency during an X-ray examination
and so should be familiar with the drugs and equipment which are kept
ready in the department. It is always wise to be aware of what might go
wrong and to have thought out beforehand what one would do if it did.

3

The Medical Laboratory

This chapter consists of three sections. The first is on handling of specimens, from safety aspects to making a blood film. The second is a table of laboratory investigations, an alphabetical list of most tests mentioning appropriate containers, volume of specimen required, concentration levels, short comments on their significance and an introduction pointing out some of the fallacies. The final section on diagnostic tests gives more details for some tests and describes a few of the dynamic procedures which assist diagnosis.

The advice given will be enhanced by a considerate and flexible approach to the individual patient and by maintaining close links with the local laboratory.

COLLECTION AND HANDLING OF SPECIMENS

General advice

Take specimens as early as possible in the working day and deliver to the laboratory promptly unless instructed otherwise.

Special or urgent tests should be requested in person.

A report is of little value lying in the laboratory and pathologists and their staff make every effort to give a speedy and efficient service. However, success depends on the co-operation of those requesting the tests. Full information will avoid errors and may be relevant to the interpretation of the results. Many investigations are now tested in batches at specified times during the day, or week, and knowledge of these local arrangements will minimise delays.

Certain specimens may be collected from outpatients (but carriage must be in approved and properly labelled transport boxes) and some tests are best arranged by the laboratory.

In summary:

Get specimens to the lab. as quickly as possible;
Use the appropriate container, correctly filled and labelled;
If in doubt, contact the lab.

Blood tests

Take blood by clean venepuncture with a minimum of venestasis and, if possible, without 'hand-clenching' by the patient. Ideally only one puncture should be made and the blood should be taken as soon as possible after applying the tourniquet. If the patient is receiving i.v. infusions take the blood from the other arm. Disposable or dry sterilised syringes, or the 'Vacutainer' system, should be used. If you fail after two attempts, or the patient complains of persistent pain, this may be the moment to ask for expert advice.

Remove the needle from the syringe and expel the blood gently into the appropriate container. Forcible ejection of blood produces haemolysis. Tubes containing anticoagulant should be stoppered and then inverted several times. Do not shake.

Containers bear colour-coded labels for different anticoagulants. There are two codes in common use (British Standard 4851 does not apply to evacuated container systems):

Container	UK (BS 4851)	ISO recommendations
Plain		
(without anticoagulant)	White	Red
Sequestrene		
(EDTA)	Pink	Lavender
Lithium heparin	Orange	Green
Sodium citrate		
(for ESR)	Mauve	Black
Sodium citrate		
(for prothrombin time)	Mauve	Blue
Fluoride/oxalate	Yellow	Grey

For further details refer to the Table of Laboratory Investigations and the Diagnostic Tests section. (p 140 et seq.)

Making a blood film

Use new cleaned microscope slides. With an ear- or finger-prick obtain a drop of blood, without pressure, and place near one end of a slide. Place this slide on a firm table with the blood drop upwards. Then put the narrow edge of another slide close to the drop of blood at an angle of about 40 degrees to the slide on the table. Draw back the top slide to make contact with the drop of blood and when the blood has spread between the slides move the top slide forward in a smooth action, maintaining the angle. Quickly dry by waving slide about.

Write the patient's name on the slide; this can be done in pencil if one edge of the slide is frosted.

With experience an even film can be obtained by slightly varying the angle of the spreader slide. The commonest error is to use too large a drop of blood. Films from venous blood may be prepared using a drop from the syringe or from mixed sequestrenated blood, taken within two hours.

Thick film preparations for malaria and filariasis require three small drops of fresh blood to be spread (not stirred) quickly and evenly over a slide to cover an area about 1 cm in diameter. Do not make the films too thick. It should be possible to read news print clearly through them. Dry thoroughly.

24-hour urine collections

It is desirable that the patient be given detailed instructions on how to make the collection (*see p* 77), stressing that voids wholly or partly lost or those added outside the exact timed period will render the test useless. The patient starts the collection after emptying the bladder completely and discarding all of this urine. The time and date should be noted on the bottle label. From this point onwards, for exactly 24 hours, all urine should be saved in the container provided and the collection finished by emptying the bladder again, but this time including the urine in the collection. Again note the time and date on the bottle label. Send to the laboratory promptly.

It is doubtful if the urinary creatinine excretion is sufficiently constant to justify its use as a reference for the excretion rate of other substances, but to express the measured excretion per mmol of urinary creatinine is an approach used when a 24-hour collection is incomplete.

The laboratory will supply any special container required. For some investigations the addition of an acid preservative is necessary. The patient should be notified not to spill or splash it. The container should be clearly labelled.

If part of a 24-hour urine specimen is separated a note must be made of the total 24-hour urine volume. The urine output at 1 year old is about 450 ml, at 4 years old 650 ml and 1500 ml in the adult.

Labelling of specimens

Before taking blood ask the patient to confirm the personal details on the request form. The date of birth is a better aid to recognition than the age.

When a patient is unfit or unable to provide identification the ward nurse, or other suitable person, must be asked to identify him. Always check the details on the inpatient identity bracelet.

Label the container, surname first, in capital letters, after adding the specimen and before leaving the patient. Whenever possible, and always when available in the case of specimens for blood grouping and cross-matching, the patient's hospital number or address should be used.

In the case of specimens for culture, for plasma glucose, cortisol and other constituents which show nyctohemeral variations of level, or when there is a series of specimens, note on the container the date and time when the specimen was taken.

Emergency service

All major laboratories run an on-call emergency service. It is costly and usually limited in scope so only use it when an investigation is essential for the patient's immediate treatment and cannot be deferred.

A sequestrene sample for a haemoglobin estimation and an examination of the blood film will often provide all the information required. A sample of plain blood taken at the same time will enable most follow-up investigations to be performed, although many laboratories prefer a heparin sample for urea and electrolytes.

For a blood glucose screen a glucose oxidase strip reading (Dextrostix-Ames p 75) is sometimes adequate but it is advisable to check the result especially in the lower range. If there is any delay a specimen in fluoride-oxalate is essential.

Keeping specimens overnight

Prompt delivery is advisable for most bacteriological examinations and is essential for amoebae in stools, trichomonads in vaginal swabs and for blood cultures. *Neisseria gonorrhoeae* swabs require transport media.

Haematological specimens are best tested at once, but haemoglobin estimations, red and white cell counts, the ESR (sedimentation rate) and platelet counts can be made on blood kept for up to 12 hours at 4°C in glass containers and anticoagulated with sequestrene. Blood films keep well.

Plasma for electrolytes should be separated at once and will then keep until the next day in the refrigerator. Some hormones are rapidly destroyed in whole blood and it is essential that plasma from such samples is separated as a matter of urgency and stored at –20°C until assayed. Do not put whole blood in the deep freeze.

Urine for biochemistry and microscopy may be kept overnight in the refrigerator without much change. If kept longer cells disintegrate, casts disappear and crystals may form. For bacteriological investigation a fresh specimen is preferable; when this is not possible the urine should be refrigerated at 4°C until cultured.

Cell counts and protein estimations are satisfactory on cerebrospinal fluid kept for a few hours in a refrigerator. For glucose estimation a little fresh c.s.f. should be placed in a fluoride-oxalate tube.

Transmission of specimens

Specimens should be sent in the appropriate container. Avoid leakage which will invalidate the result and be a health hazard to the postal and laboratory staff.

Most laboratories arrange their own despatch of specimens but if you have to arrange for a specimen to go by post to another laboratory the Post Office Guide contains full regulations. In general specimens should be sent by letter post in a sealed receptacle in an approved box, packed with sufficient material to absorb any leakage, and marked, 'Fragile with care' and 'Pathology specimen'. Be sure to enclose a letter or request form.

In certain instances it is important that deep frozen specimens do not thaw. Seek advice about packing and it may be desirable to send these specimens by one of the special services available, such as Railex, passenger train Red Star Parcel Service or Securicor.

Many laboratories use the Supra Regional Assay Service for newly developed, technically difficult and infrequently used tests. Arrangements should be made with the chemical pathologist of your own laboratory. He will know of any special collection requirements stipulated by the reference laboratory.

Safety

When handling blood or body fluids, there is always some danger of infection with an agent of serum hepatitis (such as virus B). This is more likely if the skin is damaged or the eye contaminated.

It is wise to wear protective gloves. Any contaminated part should be washed at once with copious amounts of water or saline. Spillages should be wiped with 10 per cent formalin solution or, if on a non-metallic surface, freshly diluted 1 per cent hypochlorite solution. Any contaminated equipment or fabric should be autoclaved, if possible, or soaked in hypochlorite before laundering.

Dangerous reservoirs of infection are patients known to have serum hepatitis or to have hepatitis-associated antigen in the plasma; patients with jaundice of uncertain origin; drug addicts; persons with a history of serum hepatitis; patients with Down's syndrome from institutions, and patients with chronic liver disease or chronic uraemia (especially if they have had haemodialysis in hospital).

Precautions should also be taken when dealing with a patient given a provisional diagnosis of smallpox, and with brucella, anthrax and salmonella and some tropical infections. The advice of the local consultant microbiologist or the laboratory safety officer should be obtained. In the United Kingdom the Health and Safety at Work Act, 1974, regulates the safety of the working conditions for hospital staff.

Special requirements for microbiology specimens

Specimens should be taken if possible before antibiotics are given and delivered promptly to the laboratory. Details of any antibiotics given should be stated on the request form. For details of swabs and blood cultures, *see p* 97. Culture results are usually known the next day and sensitivities to antibiotics 24 hours later. A 'direct sensitivity' can sometimes be arranged when the result is available with the culture.

Urine
A fresh midstream specimen taken directly into a wide mouthed sterile container is required. For technique, *see pp* 76 *and* 77).

Suprapubic aspiration, or bag collection, may be indicated in young children.

When a urinary tract infection is confirmed it is important to arrange further examinations after a course of treatment.

Examination for tubercule bacilli is best performed on three consecutive early morning samples. Collect all the first specimen of urine passed.

Sputum
Send the first specimen of the morning before eating or teeth cleaning and ensure it is not just saliva.

Anaerobic cultures
If an adequate amount of pus is available fill a sterile container, otherwise aspirate into a syringe using a wide-bore needle and replace this with a sealed butt before sending the labelled syringe to the laboratory without delay. With small amounts of material take paired swabs and place one in transport media. It is essential that specimens are taken from the depths of the lesion.

Mycology investigations
These usually consist of skin, nail or hair. They may be wrapped in a small piece of black paper, properly labelled and sent, by post if necessary, in an envelope. For specimens such as sputum, pus or biopsy material, collect into a sterile container and deliver to the laboratory in the usual way.

Virus investigations
Material for virus isolation should be collected as early as possible in the illness. Standard faecal specimens are suitable. From other sites (except smallpox) swabs broken off into a bottle containing transport medium (obtainable from the laboratory) should be used.

Cerebrospinal fluid should be collected in a sterile container.

It is advisable to transport specimens in an insulated box containing ice with the specimen in a securely closed plastic bag.

In cases of suspected smallpox the community physician should be consulted before collection (*p* 113).

Serological tests in microbiology

Bacterial infections. It is desirable to demonstrate a significant rise in antibody titre and, therefore, two specimens should be taken, the first as early as possible and the second usually about the third week of the illness. In the case of Widal tests details of TAB inoculations should be supplied.

Virus infections. Serological tests are used for the following infections: influenza, mumps, psittacosis-lymphogranuloma venereum, adenovirus, respiratory syncytial virus, herpes simplex, mycoplasma, Q fever, measles and rubella. Full details should be given including the date of onset, any rashes or enlarged lymph nodes, vaccination history and antibiotic therapy. In all requests for viral tests it is important to state the virus considered most likely to be the cause of the illness.

Special requirements for histology specimens

Tissues to be examined fresh ('frozen sections') must arrive at the laboratory in a plain container within minutes of taking. Arrangements should be made with the laboratory beforehand.

Routine specimens are placed in wide mouthed containers holding formol saline ten times the volume of the specimen. On no account should tissues be allowed to dry. Most departments supply containers of various sizes filled with formol saline. Certain tissues (*e.g.* testicular biopsy) are usually fixed in Bouin's solution.

For some histochemistry tests formol saline is contraindicated, so check with your own laboratory, which will also be able to supply details of requirements for preservation and transport of tissue enzyme specimens to the Supra Regional Assay Service when assistance is needed in the diagnosis of inherited metabolic disease.

Sputum diagnosis
Send a fresh specimen, as for microbiology, on three consecutive days but not within seven days after bronchoscopy.

Ascitic and pleural fluids
Send a plain specimen and one in a container with 3.8 per cent sodium citrate (1 ml/25 ml of fluid).

Gastric washings
Determine any special requirements from your laboratory first. On the day before the test no food is allowed after 1900 h or fluid after midnight. At 0700 h on the day of the test give a mouth wash and check that dentures have been removed. Pass a Ryle's tube (which has an extra large hole at the end) preferably via the mouth (*p* 99). After aspirating gastric juice give 250 ml of isosmotic sodium chloride solution. Elevate the foot of the bed and encourage the patient to change posture while aspirating. Send the resting juice and aspirate to the laboratory.

Urine
Collect 50 ml of early morning urine and deliver to the laboratory for examination within six hours. If there is likely to be delay the early morning specimen should be passed into a suitable container in which there is 50 ml of methylated spirit.

Cervical and vaginal cytology
Some training is needed before taking the smears. (*see p* 98). Ideally take the smear in midcycle and before a manual examination is carried out.

Smear both sides of the Ayre's spatula (*p* 98) evenly on a glass slide, with one stroke from each, and immediately plunge the slide into the ether and alcohol fixative, or apply the bottle fixative immediately while the smear is wet. After fixing and drying (allow 30 minutes) the slides should be sent in the container provided together with a completed cervical cytology request/report form. If there is any question of uterine malignancy a smear from a vaginal aspirate is required and for information regarding hormone studies a smear from the lateral vaginal wall is required.

Vaccines and antisera

Immunoglobulin, antivaccinial immunoglobulins, anti-Au immunoglobulins, rabies vaccine and antisera and typhus vaccine are issued by many Public Health Laboratories. In Britain material for immunisation against diphtheria, tuberculosis (BCG) pertussis, poliomyelitis, tetanus, measles, rubella, cholera and typhoid (either monovalent or combined with paratyphoid A and B) is obtainable from the department of the community physician or commercially. Yellow fever vaccine must be used within 30 minutes of exposure to room temperature and so it is only available at certain centres and some air terminals.

Drugs and laboratory tests

Many drugs interfere with laboratory tests either by causing changes in the tissues or for technical reasons in doing the test. Fluorimetric methods for determining plasma cortisol will give erroneously high results if the patient is taking fusidic acid, mepacrine or spironolactone. Reducing methods for the determination of glucose will be unreliable if the body fluid contains large amounts of reducing agents such as ascorbic and nalidixic acid. Drugs often cause urine to be abnormally coloured. The technique of collection may be important. Skin swabbing with spirit must be avoided in alcohol tests and syringes lubricated with glycerine must not be used in triglyceride determinations. Other examples are mentioned in the Table of Laboratory Investigations (*p* 142 *et seq.*). If in doubt consult the laboratory.

TABLE OF LABORATORY INVESTIGATIONS

Specimen containers. Specimens need to be collected in the appropriate containers for valid results. Specimens for determination of the glucose level are usually collected into an inhibitor of glycolysis, such as sodium fluoride. These fluoride/oxalate containers are obviously not suitable for other tests, *e.g.* sodium and some enzymes. Sodium and potassium can be tested using either serum (collected in the plain container and allowed to clot) or plasma (collected in a lithium heparin container); which is required depends on the local laboratory arrangements. Needless to add, lithium heparin containers are unsuitable for serum lithium tests; these are usually collected into a plain tube. Many haematology investigations require whole blood collected into a suitable anticoagulant which does not distort the cells, *e.g.* sequestrene (EDTA). For some blood constituents, such as urea, there is only a slight difference between the level for whole blood and that in the plasma or serum. Urate shows significantly different levels for whole blood and for serum, while for potassium the whole blood and plasma levels are so different that it is essential to avoid haemolysis. Sometimes the anticoagulant required is determined by the method of assay and will, therefore, vary from laboratory to laboratory.

Volume of specimen. The volume of body fluid required for a test may vary depending on the method of assay. For example, if serum vitamin B_{12} is determined by bioassay, about 10 ml of blood is required; if by radioimmunoassay less than 2 ml is required. The volume of plasma or serum available will also depend on the haematocrit of the blood and if multiple tests are required on the same specimen it is seldom necessary to take as much blood as would be required for single tests done on separate occasions.

Reference value. A normal range is established by statistical treatment of data obtained from a large population sample. The aim is to provide a range of values within which lie 95 per cent of normal individuals. Even by this criterion 1 in 20 of normal individuals will have a value outside the normal range. Values also depend on the population sample; the age, sex, diet, whether ambulant or bedridden and also on the type of specimen and the method used for the test. There may be more than one normal range for any constituent and ideally the method of assay should always be stated. Some ranges are arbitrary because there is inadequate knowledge of the population distribution. The doctor should satisfy himself about the 'normal range' for his patients and for his laboratory. The 'Reference value' provided refers to ambulant adult outpatients unless stated otherwise.

The values for many blood constituents vary during a 24-hour period. This applies especially to certain hormones such as cortisol but many other substances show changes and the time of day also affects certain function tests, *e.g.* glucose tolerance tests.

The drug concentrations and the therapeutic ranges quoted do not take into account factors such as age, coexisting disease and administration of other drugs which could modify the individual response.

Unit nomenclature. The SI system is based on the metric system and has seven fundamental (or base) units of measurement. They include the metre (m) for length; the kilogram (kg) for mass; the second (s) for time and the mole (mol) for amount of substance. Combinations of these produce derived units, *e.g.* concentration can be measured in mol/m^3 and prefixes to indicate fractions or multiples of the units have also been recommended. Prefixes commonly used in medicine are:

Factor	Prefix	Symbol
10^{-1}	deci-	d
10^{-2}	centi-	c
10^{-3}	milli-	m
10^{-6}	micro-	μ
10^{-9}	nano-	n
10^{-12}	pico-	p
10^{-15}	femto-	f

e.g. 0.000001 g = 10^{-6} g = 1 μg

To convert from mmol/1 to mg/dl:

$$\frac{\text{Concentration (mmol/1)} \times \text{Molecular weight}}{10}$$

In the table a conversion factor to multiply from old to SI units is provided for the commonly used tests. Where the molecular weight cannot be determined, *e.g.* globulin, the analysis is reported as weight per litre.

Enzymes-nomenclature and units of measurement. Each enzyme has the Enzyme Commission number, *e.g.* glutamic oxaloacetic transaminase (GOT) is EC 2.6.6.1., renamed L-aspartate: 2-oxoglutarate aminotransferase, the trivial name being aspartate aminotransferase (ATT or AST). Enzymes are measured by the rate at which a reaction proceeds and recommended units of activity (such as International Units/1 or Katal/1) are not yet fully adopted. It is important to remember that values of enzyme activity which vary by fourfold may still be expressed as the same unit depending on conditions such as substrate and temperature of assay. Each doctor must be prepared to find out whether the laboratories which he is using are measuring enzymes by identical methods and if not he must make himself conversant with the values which refer to his patients.

Urine preservatives. If required refrigeration or the addition of 10 ml of 2g/dl boric acid will serve for most chemical analyses, unless otherwise stated.

Systems key: U = urine, B = blood, S = serum, P = plasma, Erys = erythrocytes, c.s.f. = cerebrospinal fluid, Lks = leucocytes, F = faeces

System	Test	Container	Volume	Reference value	Remarks
U	Abnormal pigments	Plain	20 ml	Negative	Pink/red urines can occur in porphyria, phenindione therapy and, in some patients, after eating beetroot. Dark brown/black urines are seen in paroxysmal myoglobinuria, after i.v. iron, during methyl dopa and L-dopa therapy and in alkaptonuria. Blood can give a red or smoky brown colour. Green/blue urines are usually due to methylene blue (from sweets or pills). In jaundice urine can be yellow, brown or green. Other causes of yellow/orange urine include tetracycline therapy and taking phenolphthalein
S	Acetone	Plain	10 ml	50–400 μmol/l (0.3–2.0 mg/dl)	*See* Ketones
U	Acetylator phenotype	Plain	20 ml	The urine is collected on second day after two days of sulphasalazine 500 mg bd. Some drugs (isoniazid, sulphonamides, hydralazine, phenelzine) are polymorphically acetylated in man. Slow and rapid acetylators are found	

System	Test	Container	Volume	Reference value	Remarks
S	Acid phosphatase (ACP 3.1.3.2)	Plain	5 ml	0–4 U/l (0–3 King Armstrong Units/dl) Formol stable (prostatic) or tartrate inhibited.	Raised level (often 5–50 times normal) in prostatic carcinoma with metastases. Level falls on successful treatment of the tumour. Level can be altered during urinary retention and after rectal examination. Haemolysis should be avoided. Separate serum within 2 h. Total acid phosphatase level may be raised in Paget's disease of bone, and with carcinomatous metastases in bone (over 7 U/l)
P	ACTH	Heparin (plastic)	15 ml	See Adrenal-pituitary function tests in Diagnostic Tests section. *p* 207	
	Actinomycosis	Plain sterile	Specimen of pus		
	Acromegaly			See Adrenal-pituitary function tests *p* 210	
	Addison's disease			See Adrenal-pituitary function tests *p* 206	
	Adenovirus			Throat swab in viral transport media, paired sera, conjunctival swab, faeces	
S	Alanine aminotransferase (GPT, ALT 2.6.1.2)	Plain	5 ml	2–15 U/l	Levels raised in necrosis of liver or heart cells. Avoid haemolysis

System	Test	Container	Volume	Reference value	Remarks
S	Albumin	Plain	10 ml	30–50 g/l	Low in chronic liver cirrhosis, nephrosis, malabsorption and enteropathy. Bisalbuminaemia and analbuminaemia are rare inherited conditions (Note prealbumin range 0.2–0.4 g/l)
B	Alcohol (ethanol)	Fluoride-oxalate	2 ml	Legal limit 80 mg/dl (17.4 mmol/l)	Do not use an alcohol skin swab. Urine concentration about one-third higher than in blood. Fatal level about 500 mg/dl (or 5.0 g/l)
S	Aldolase (ALS 4.1.2.13)	Plain	5 ml	2–7 U/l	Avoid haemolysis. Increased in muscle disease, (e.g. Duchenne type dystrophy) hepatitis, some anaemias and malignancy. Seldom provides more information than other enzymes. See Creatine kinase
P	Aldosterone	Heparin	10 ml	85–850 pmol/l (Patient at rest. Verify normal range with own laboratory)	Should be separated and despatched on the day it is taken. Of value in investigation of Conn's syndrome and secondary aldosteronism, but only indicated if patients have hypertension and hypokalaemia. Administration of metopirone, diuretics, purgatives and oestrogens should be discontinued for three weeks beforehand. See Renin

System	Test	Container	Volume	Reference value	Remarks
Lks	Alkaline phosphatase	Sequestrene (with 4 fresh blood films)	5 ml	25–100 (score/100 neutrophils)	Raised in leucocytosis. Reduced in myeloid leukaemia
S	Alkaline phosphatase (ALP 3.1.3.1)	Plain	5 ml	20–90 U/l (3–13 KA units/dl)	Level may be more than doubled in children. Increased in pregnancy, in bone diseases, in biliary obstruction and primary biliary cirrhosis and primary hyperparathyroidism with associated bone disease. Decreased in hypophosphatasaemia
U	Alkaptonuria	Plain	5 ml	Homogentisic acid found in urine	An inborn error of metabolism
	Alpha-1-antitrypsin	(See α_1-Antitrypsin)			
P	Amino acid nitrogen	Heparin	5 ml	2.5–4.0 mmol/l	Changes in amino acid metabolism only reflected to a limited extent by the plasma levels. Raised in renal failure and hepatic necrosis
U	Amino Acid Nitrogen	100 ml 1 mol/l HCl	24 h	4–20 mmol/24 h	See Hydroxyproline and Amino aciduria
U	Amino aciduria		20 ml		Early morning specimen. Excess amino acids due to increased plasma levels or tubular defects. May be genetic, e.g. phenylketonuria or secondary to liver disease

System	Test	Container	Volume	Reference value	Remarks
U	Aminolaevulate (o-aminolaevulinate)	With 25 ml 6 mol/1 HCl	24 h	1–40 μmol/24 h (0–5.3 mg/24 h)	Increased amounts in acute intermittent porphyria. May excrete 750 μmol/24 h. Note. Urine darkens only on standing
Erys	δ-Aminolaevulinate dehydratase (4.2.1.24)	Heparin	2 ml	(Verify with own lab)	Keep refrigerated. Decreased activity in lead poisoning. Too sensitive a test for routine use
P	Amitriptyline (and Nortriptyline)	Heparin	20 ml		Therapeutic range 100–200 μg/1 Severe overdose at 1000 μg/1
P	Ammonium	Heparin	10 ml (arrange with Laboratory)	11–45 μmol/1 (20–75 μg/dl)	Deliver to laboratory immediately
U	Ammonium		24 h	20–70 mmol/24 h	After ammonium chloride load test the rate of ammonium excretion is low in renal disease. Infected urines may give abnormal results
	Amniotic fluid bilirubin	Protect container from light	10 ml	Less than 0.4 (mg/g) Less than 6.5 (μmol/g)	Bilirubin to protein ratio enables prediction of neonatal haemolysis. Bilirubin levels elevated in haemolytic disease

System	Test	Container	Volume	Reference value	Remarks
Amniotic fluid (continued)	α_1-Fetoprotein	(not blood-stained)	5 ml	2000–20000 $\mu g/l$ maximum at 17 weeks (less than 5 $\mu g/l$ at delivery)	Raised levels have increased incidence of neural tube defects
	L/S ratio				Lecithin/sphingomyelin ratio for assessment of foetal lung maturity. Maturation associated with lecithin increase. The ratio is greater than 2.0 at 36–40 weeks
	tissue enzymes	Sterile			Obtain at 15/16 week gestation for diagnosis of inherited metabolic diseases
	chromosomal abnormalities	Sterile plastic			Amniotic fluid can be used for antenatal detection *See* chromosomal analysis
S	Amoebiasis (*E. histolytica*)	Plain	5 ml		Immunofluorescent test positive (often over 1/200) in most patients. Negative test advised before steroids in *e.g.* ulcerative colitis
F	Amoebic dysentery	Fresh specimen (keep warm)			Trophozoites usually only found if blood in the stool
U	Amphetamine	Plain	50 ml		Can be detected days after ingestion

System	Test	Container	Volume	Reference value	Remarks
S	Amylase (AMS 3.2.1.1)	Plain	5 ml	Less than 300 iu/l (60–160 Somogyi units/dl)	Usually over 1000 iu/l in acute pancreatitis. Level shows some increase in mumps and penetrating peptic ulcer. Isoenzymes are more specific
U	Amylase		24 h	200–1500 U/24 h	After pancreatitis level may remain increased longer than in serum
	Amyloidosis				Deposition of abnormal proteins in conditions of immunological incompetence. Diagnosis can be confirmed by rectal biopsy
	Anencephaly			See α_1-Fetoprotein	
B	Antenatal pregnancy routine (Hb, VDRL, Group, Rh antibodies)	Plain, and sequestrene	10 ml 2 ml		
	Anthrax	Material from the local lesion		Obtain advice of local microbiologist first	
B	Antibodies	Plain	5 ml	Negative	See tests, e.g. Antinuclear factors
	Anticoagulant therapy			See Prothrombin time	Note drug interactions. Barbiturates and other sedatives, antibiotics, salicylates and other anti-inflammatory agents, phenylbutazone, clofibrate, cholestyramine and steroids

System	Test	Container	Volume	Reference value	Remarks
S	Anti-DNA	Plain	5 ml		Various types described. Presence usually associated with severe cases of systemic lupus erythematosus in the presence of renal involvement and low serum complement values. Often normal in drug-induced SLE
S	Antinuclear factors	Plain	5 ml		Titres greater than 1/100 are found in systemic lupus erythematosus. A negative test virtually excludes SLE. Raised titres also found in chronic (lupoid) hepatitis
S	α_1-Antitrypsin	Plain	5 ml	0.9–5.0g/l (usually about 2 g/l)	Congenital deficiency associated with early development of emphysema and neonatal hepatitis. Homozygote ZZ most affected. It is an acute phase protein, so test when patient not ill with an infection
U	Arsenic		24 h	Less than 0.67 μmol/l (less than 50 μg/l)	
	Ascitic fluid				In general the findings are exudate (protein over 3 g/dl, often clots, many cells—leucocytes, culture may be positive) and transudate (protein less than 2 g/dl, no fibrin, and glucose level as in blood)
Lks	Ascorbate	Heparin	5 ml	115–345 nmol/10^8 (21–53 μg/10^8) leucocytes or 1.3–2.5 mmol/l	Provides best indication of body vitamin C. Some methods require special sequestrene containers. Check with your laboratory

System	Test	Container	Volume	Reference value	Remarks
P	Ascorbate	Heparin	5 ml	35–90 μmol/l (0.6–1.6 mg/dl)	Plasma levels reflect turnover
U	Ascorbate	If delay add 10 ml glacial acetic acid			Collect 2-hour urine sample commencing 4 hours after 700 mg of ascorbic acid orally. At saturation should contain more than 30 mg of ascorbic acid. Specimen should be sent to the laboratory immediately. Patients with deficiency take more than 3 days to reach saturation.
S	ASO (anti-streptolysin titre)	Plain	5 ml	50–200 units/ml	Less than 50 u/ml virtually excludes acute rheumatism. High values are found following streptococcal infections
S	Aspartate aminotransferase (GOT, AST 2.6.1.1)	Plain	5 ml	5–20 U/l	Levels increased after cardiac infarction within 6–18 h to reach a maximum 1 to 2 days later, returning to normal by 5 days. With a minor infarct the peak may only reach the upper limit of normal. Also increased in hepatic necrosis, even before jaundice appears. Slight elevation after pulmonary emboli and intake of alcohol. Avoid haemolysis
B	Australia antigen/antibody	Plain (screw cap)	2 ml	Negative	Usually positive in patients with acute serum hepatitis (virus B). Handle specimens with care

System	Test	Container	Volume	Reference value	Remarks
B	Barbiturate	Heparin or plain	10 ml		Significance of level depends on subtype. Wide individual variation, and alcohol has additive effect. Fatal coma may occur at 3 mg/dl, or less, of short acting type and 9 mg/dl of long acting type. To convert mg/dl to μmol/l multiply by 54.29 or divide by 0.0184, (taking mol. wt. of diethylbarbituric acid as 184). *See* Phenobarbitone for therapeutic levels
B	Base Excess	Heparinised syringe	5 ml	-2 to +2 mmol/l	*See* Blood pH and Gas determinations *p* 217
U	Bence Jones protein	Plain	50 ml		The light chains of certain immunoglobulins. The urine usually needs to be concentrated. Found in many patients with myeloma. Early morning specimen preferred
P	Bicarbonate (plasma)	Heparin	5 ml	21–31 mmol/l	The total concentration of bicarbonates and carbonates
P	Bicarbonate (standard)			21–26 mmol/l	The concentration of bicarbonate from fully oxygenated whole blood at 37°C and a PCO_2 of 5.3 kPa. *See* Blood pH and Gas determinations *p* 216
S	Bile acids	Plain	10 ml	0.3–2.5 mg/dl	
U	Bile pigments	Plain	20 ml		Normally no detectable bilirubin and small amounts of urobilinogen. Bilirubin appears early in hepatocellular disease and cholestasis. Urobilinogen increased in haemolytic anaemia. May disappear with complete obstruction

System	Test	Container	Volume	Reference value	Remarks
S	Bilirubin (total)	Plain	5ml	5–17 μmol/l (0.3–1.0 mg/dl) (Conversion factor for traditional to SI units: 17.1, expressing conjugated bilirubin as bilirubin)	The conjugated fraction usually less than 4 μmol/l (0.2 mg/dl). In haemolytic anaemia unconjugated bilirubin increased. In hepatocellular disease and cholestasis usually conjugated bilirubin level increased. Seldom of diagnostic value because most cases are mixed
B	Bleeding time				Observe the flow of blood from an ear-prick on to blotting paper and note the time when the bleeding ceases. Normal values are between 2 and 7 minutes. See Clotting deficiency tests
B	Blood count				see Haemoglobin, leucocytes, MCH, red blood cell (RBC) count and reticulocytes
B	Blood culture				5 ml asceptically directly into two or three culture bottles as advised by the local microbiologist. (See Clinical procedures p 97). If the culture is negative this will be reported after a week
B	Blood gases			PCO_2 4.5–6.1 kPa (34–46 mmHg) PO_2 10.6–13.2 kPa (80–100 mmHg)	See Blood pH and Gas determinations p 215 (Arterial gas tensions may also be written $PaCO_2$ or PaO_2)
B	Blood-grouping and cross-matching	Plain	10 ml		For routine surgical requests at least 24 hours notice is advisable. 2 ml of blood in a sequestrene container for haemoglobin is suggested
B	Blood volume (mean)			Men 69 ml/kg Women 65 ml/kg	Range 65–100 ml/kg or 2.5–4.0 litres/m^2 of body surface. Both blood and plasma volume increase in pregnancy to a maxima at 32 weeks

System	Test	Container	Volume	Reference value	Remarks
	Bone Marrow (consult haematologist)				
B	Bromide	Plain	5 ml	0.8–1.5 mg/dl	Symptoms appear at 100 mg/dl, some individual variation
B	Brucella antibodies	Plain	5 ml	Less than 1/80	Blood cultures and serum for antibodies should be taken before a Brucellin skin test is performed. Titre of 1/40 Brucella C/F test suggests active infection
S	BSP (bromosulphthalein excretion test)	Plain	10 ml	Less than 1.5 mg/dl retained at 25 min and 0.5 mg/dl at 45 min	With patient fasting, inject i.v. 5 mg/kg BSP slowly. Ensure injection not outside the vein. Have anaphylaxis tray ready. Proteinuria should not be present
P	BUN (Blood urea nitrogen)	Heparin or plain	5 ml	8–18 mg/dl	See Urea. (BUN value multiplied by 2.14 gives urea value in mg/dl)
S	B₁₂ (see folate)	Plain sterile	15 ml (allows for folate and repeat if required) less if RIA methods used	160–925 ng/l (conversion factor for pmol/l is 0.738)	Reduced in megaloblastic intrinsic factor deficiency anaemia and in some malabsorption syndromes. High levels in myeloproliferative disorders. Some methods may be affected by the presence of antibiotics in the serum. Bacterial contamination may raise the level

System	Test	Container	Volume	Reference value	Remarks
S	Caeruloplasmin	Plain	5 ml	0.2–0.5 g/l (200–500 mg/l)	An α_2 globulin. Contains most of the serum copper. Decreased in Wilson's disease and nephrosis. Low in neonates. Raised in pregnancy
P	Calcitonin	Heparin	10 ml	Fasting less than 50 pg/ml (verify normal range with own laboratory)	Centrifuge immediately and store plasma at –20°C. Transfer deep frozen. Liaise with reference laboratory. (Physiological antagonist to parathyroid hormone)
S	Calcium (total)	Plain (glass)	5 ml	2.12–2.60 mmol/l (8.5–10.5 mg/dl) (conversion factor 0.25) At birth 1.9–3.0 mmol/l (ionised calcium 1.03–1.23 mmol/l)	Take in fasting state and with minimum of venestasis. Raised in hyperparathyroidism (often intermittently) hypervitaminosis D. Also in neonates, milk-alkali syndrome, myelomatosis (and other neoplasms) and sarcoidosis. Reduced in hypoparathyroidism, malabsorption, renal disease. Ionised fraction (about 50%) is of most importance physiologically. It is reduced in tetany
F	Calcium		1–5 day	100–200 mmol/kg (400–800 mg/24 h)	Balance studies provide information about the progression of disorders such as osteoporosis
U	Calcium		24 h	On average diet 2.5–7.5 mmol/24h (100–300 mg/24h). Conversion factor 0.025	Raised in hypercalcaemia and idiopathic hypercalciuria. See Kidney function tests p 219

System	Test	Container	Volume	Reference value	Remarks
U	Cannabis		10 ml		Severe psychosis associated with levels over 100 $\mu g/l$
P	Carbon dioxide (total) TCO_2	Heparin	5 ml	21–31 mmol/l	Increased in airway obstructive disease. Reduced in diabetic acidosis. A measurement of bicarbonate and free CO_2
B	Carboxyhaemoglobin (carbon monoxide poisoning)	Heparin	5 ml	Less than 0.03 (3%)	Heavy smokers may have 8%. Up to 20% can occur in unfavourable conditions of atmospheric pollution. Coma at 50%. 70% and over usually fatal. Full container if possible
P	Carbamazepine	Heparin	5 ml	3–13 mg/l	Usual therapeutic range
S	Carcinoembryonic antigen (CEA)	Plain	5 ml	Less than 3 $\mu g/l$	Over 20 $\mu g/l$ suggestive of cancer of colon or bronchus, pancreas, breast. No use for early detection, mainly for follow up of colonic tumours
	Carcinoid	(See 5-Hydroxyindole acetate)			
P	β-carotene	Heparin	10 ml	0.9–5.6 $\mu mol/l$ (50–300 $\mu g/dl$)	Precursor of vitamin A. May be decreased in malabsorption and increased in hypothyroidism
P	Catecholamines	Heparin	20 ml	Less than 5 nmol/l (1 $\mu g/l$). (adrenaline/noradrenaline)	Increased after shock, some drugs and with phaeochromocytoma

System	Test	Container	Volume	Reference value	Remarks
U	Catecholamines	25 ml 6 mol/l HCl	24 h	0.05–0.55 μmol/24 h (10–100 μg/24 h) as adrenaline	Comprise dopamine, adrenaline and noradrenaline. Rapidly removed from the blood, 5% excreted unchanged, rest as metabolites. See HMMA, and Metadrenaline
c.s.f.	Cerebrospinal fluid (routine)	The main part in sterile plain containers Some in fluoride-oxalate			See Cerebrospinal fluid in Diagnostic tests p 211
S	C1 Esterase Inhibitor	Plain	5 ml	0.15–0.35 g/l	Low levels associated with hereditary angioneurotic oedema
P	Chloride	Heparin	5 ml	95–105 mmol/l	Increased in hyperchloraemic acidosis, after transplantation of ureters. Decreased in salt depletion
U	Chloride		24 h	100–250 mmol/24 h	Normally equals dietary intake
Sweat	Chloride	(See Sodium)			
S	Cholesterol	Plain or sequestrene	5 ml	3.6–7.2 mmol/l (140–275 mg/dl) About 75% esterified	Increased in nephrosis, cholestasis, cretinism and in type II and III hyperlipidaemias. Exogenous origin from meat and egg yolk. Synthesised in liver, source of steroids and bile acids. Lower levels in children. See Lipoprotein investigations in the Diagnostic Tests section p 220

System	Test	Container	Volume	Reference value	Remarks
S	Cholinesterase (pseudocholinesterase CHE, CHS 3.1.1.8)	Plain (or heparin or sequestrene)	5 ml	0.6–1.3 µmol/min/ml varies with method (8–18 U/l) dibucaine number about 80, fluoride no. 60	Decreased in organophosphorus poisoning and other acquired conditions. Genetic variants have reduced activity, some are recognised by a dibucaine or fluoride number of 10–30. Such cases are extremely sensitive to suxamethonium and have prolonged apnoea
B	Chromosomal Analysis	Heparin (sterile) 2 ml Verify with own laboratory			For microcultures 0.2–0.4 ml straight into culture medium. May require marrow specimen, amniotic fluid or, where mosaicism is suspected, tissue. Results of karyotyping available after 48 h (marrow), 14 days (blood), longer for amniotic fluid and tissue
B	Clotting deficiency tests	Citrate 2 x 2 ml Plain 2 x 5 ml Sequestrene 2 ml (verify with own laboratory)		Prothrombin Time (usually about 11–14 secs)	Compare with control. Of value in phenindione and warfarin anticoagulant therapy. Prolonged in Factor I, II, V, VII and X deficiency. (Often reported as a ratio. Usual therapeutic range of 2.0–2.5)
				Kaolin-cephalin clotting time/partial thromboplastin time	Compare with control. A test for Factor VIII. Prolonged in Factor I, II, V, VIII, IX, XI, XII deficiency

System	Test	Container	Volume	Reference value	Remarks
Clotting deficiency tests (continued)				Thrombin time (about 5 secs)	Compare with control. A test for fibrinogen (Factor I)
				Bleeding time (2-7 minutes Ivy)	Compare with control. A test for platelet and vascular endothelium function
				Fibrin degradation products (less than 40 μg/ml)	Test for fibrinolysin. Increased in intravascular coagulation
				Full blood count including platelets	These tests or those advised, should be arranged with your laboratory, which may suggest methods of assay for abnormal factors
B	Clotting time (whole blood)	Plain capillary tube		(Lee and White) 4-10 minutes	
B	PCO_2	Heparin		4.5-6.1 kPa (34-46 mmHg) Conversion factor 0.133	See Blood pH and Gas determinations pp 109 and 216
S	Cobalamin	Plain	15 ml	160-925 ng/l	See B_{12}
S	Cold agglutinins	Plain	5 ml	Less than 1/32	Proteins which agglutinate RBCs in the cold (mostly due to Anti-I specificity). May occur in lymphoma. Transient appearance associated with infections. Must be clotted and separated at 37°C

System	Test	Container	Volume	Reference value	Remarks
	Collagen	(*See* Hydroxyproline)			
S	Complement (C3)	Plain	5 ml	0.7–1.7 g/l (70–170 mg/dl)	Raised in inflammation, reduced in renal SLE
S	Complement (C4)	Plain	5 ml	0.25–0.75 g/l	Level reduced in C1 esterase inhibitor deficiency
	Conn's syndrome (*see* Aldosterone)				
B	Coombs' test (AHG)	Plain	5 ml		Note—direct anti-human globulin test shows that RBCs are coated with globulin antibodies, as in haemolytic disease of the newborn. —indirect test allow globulin antibodies to react with RBCs in vitro before adding AHG. Used to detect antibodies
S	Copper	Plain	10 ml	13–24 μmol/l (80–150 μg/dl)	Decreased in Wilson's disease (hepatolenticular degeneration), but levels vary
U	Copper		24 h	0.2–0.8 μmol/24 h (10–50 μg/24 h)	Increased in Wilson's disease. When treated with penicillamine further increase

System	Test	Container	Volume	Reference value	Remarks
B	Coproporphyrins	Heparin	20 ml	0–60 nmol/l packed erythrocytes (0–4 μg/dl)	Increased in congenital porphyria and lead poisoning
F		Suitable specimen		0–30 nmol/g (0–20 μg/g dry weight)	Increased congenital porphyria (type 1), in porphyria variegata, hereditary coproporphyria, symptomatic cutaneous hepatic and erythropoietic protoporphyria
U		Exclude light	24 h	50–350 nmol/24 h (30–220 μg/24 h)	Increased in congenital porphyria, porphyria variegata, hereditary coproporphyria, symptomatic cutaneous hepatic and lead poisoning
P	Cortisol	Heparin	5 ml	200–700 nmol/l (7–25 μg/dl) Conversion factor 27	Transcortin binding sites saturated at 700 nmol/l (25 μg/dl). Children have adult levels after one month. Values range from an average of 390 nmol/l (14.5 μg/dl) at 0800–1000 h, to less than 220 nmol/l (8 μg/dl) at 2400 h. *See* Adrenal pituitary function tests *p* 205
U	Cortisol		24 h	220–1100 nmol/24 h	The levels found depend on the method of assay and the sex of the patient. In males, if less than 335 nmol/24 h (females 280 nmol/24 h) unlikely to have Cushing's syndrome

System	Test	Container	Volume	Reference value	Remarks
S	C-Reactive protein	Plain	5 ml	Negative (less than 4 mg/l)	An α_1-globulin which appears in the serum in acute inflammatory conditions
S	Creatine	Plain	10 ml	15–45 μmol/l (0.2–0.6 mg/dl)	Increased in muscular dystrophy. Avoid haemolysis
U	Creatine		24 h	0–400 μmol/24 h (0–50 mg/24 h)	Increased in childhood, pregnancy and muscle disorders
S	Creatine kinase (CPK, CK 2.7.3.2)	Plain or sequestrene	5 ml	10–70 U/l (verify with own laboratory, lower levels in females)	Increases within 4 hours of cardiac infarction, returning to normal within 3 days. The maximum level reached may bear a direct relationship to the size of the infarct. Raised in muscular dystrophy, all diseases with damaged muscle, after exercise and even injections. The level is usually normal in liver disease
P	Creatine kinase–MB (CK–MB)	Sequestrene	5 ml	0–8 U/l	Isoenzyme of CK. After cardiac infarction activity rises within 4 h, reaches a peak about 20 h and returns to normal after two days. Not altered by liver disease. A second peak of activity suggests reinfarction
S	Creatinine	Plain or heparin	5 ml	60–120 μmol/l (0.7–1.4 mg/dl)	Raised in renal failure. Unlike urea, mainly unaffected by dietary changes

System	Test	Container	Volume	Reference value	Remarks
U	Creatinine		24 h	9–17 mmol/24 h (1–2 g/24 h)	*See* Kidney function tests *p* 217. If preservative required add 5 ml/1 of 1% aqueous merthiolate
S & U	Creatinine clearance			Test normally about 100 ml/min (1.7 ml/s)	Reduced in renal failure. *See* Kidney function tests *p* 217
B	Cross-matching	Plain 10 ml			Collect blood before giving dextran. For neonates also take sample of maternal blood. 2 ml of blood in a sequestrene container for haemoglobin is suggested
S	Cryoglobulin	Plain	5 ml (keep at 37°C)		Globulins that precipitate on cooling. Found in many conditions, *e.g.* SLE, syphilis, hepatitis, cirrhosis and leukaemia. May be mixed or monoclonal
c.s.f.	Routine	The main part in sterile plain containers. Some in fluoride-oxalate			*See* Cerebrospinal fluid in diagnostic tests *p* 211
B	Culture	Consult the local pathologist for advice as to suitable containers, media, time for taking the blood and how to deal with the specimens. *See* Blood culture			
U	Cystine and cysteine		24 h	10–100 mg/24 h	Increased with ornithine, arginine and lysine in cystinuria. Cystinuria is associated with renal stone formation (unrelated to cystinosis)

System	Test	Container	Volume	Reference value	Remarks
U	Cytomegalic inclusion disease	Add to equal volume of provided culture medium			Probably commonest congenital infection. May excrete virus for many months
B	Defibrination syndrome	Citrate Sequestrene Plain	9 ml 2 ml 5 ml	See Fibrinogen	May occur as a complication of intrauterine death, thoracic operations, carcinomatosis and incompatible blood transfusion
U	11-Deoxycortisol		24 h	Over 28 nmol/l after metyrapone (metopirone)	Increased in certain forms of congenital adrenal hyperplasia
P	Dextropropoxyphene	Heparin	5 ml		Levels of more than 1.8 mg/dl found in overdose of distalgesic, but levels variable. See Paracetamol
	Diabetes	See Glucose and Diagnostic Tests in Diabetes p 212			
P	Diazepam	Heparin	10 ml		Usual levels less than 1.0 mg/l. Severe overdose levels about 5.0 mg/l
P	Digoxin	Heparin	10 ml	1–2 ng/ml (μg/l) (1.3–2.6 nmol/l) State time of last dose	Take specimen 6–8 h after last dose of digoxin. Up to 2 ng/ml is usually safe. Under surveillance up to 3 ng/ml is unlikely to be toxic if renal function and plasma potassium satisfactory
	1,25-Dihydroxy-cholecalciferol (See vitamin D)				Level increased by action of PTH. Acts on gut to increase absorption of calcium and phosphate

System	Test	Container	Volume	Reference value	Remarks
S	Diphenylhydantoin (Epanutin, phenytoin)	Plain or heparin	5 ml		Therapeutic levels 7–17 µg/ml (7–17 mg/l)
	Diphtheria	Nose and throat swabs			Consult the pathologist. In doubtful cases a Paul-Bunnell test may be of help. The community physician's department should be informed of strongly suspected cases
S	Doriden	Plain	5 ml		Therapeutic levels less than 4 mg/l. Severe overdosage more than 30 mg/l (3 mg/dl)
U	'Drug screen' (arrange with lab)	All available urine (at least 50 ml). Keep frozen if delayed			
P	Electrolytes	Heparin	5 ml	Potassium 3.6–5.2 mmol/l Sodium 135–145 mmol/l Bicarbonate 21–31 mmol/l Chloride 95–105 mmol/l	Deliver to the laboratory within 2 h
U	Electrolytes	(See sodium, potassium, chloride)			

System	Test	Container	Volume	Reference value	Remarks
B	Enteric fever (typhoid)	Plain	10 ml (for Widal test)		Culture of blood, faeces and urine may be necessary. Give details of TAB inoculations. Discuss with consultant about notifying strongly suspected cases to the community physician's department
P	Epanutin (phenytoin)	Plain or heparin	5 ml	(See Diphenylhydantoin)	
P	Epilim	Heparin	5 ml	(See Valproate)	
B	Erythrocytes	Sequestrene	2 ml	(See Red blood cell count)	
B	ESR (erythrocyte sedimentation rate, Westergren)	Directed volume into measured citrate (or sequestrene if arranged with laboratory)		Young males up to 8 mm/h Females 12 mm/h	Increases in pregnancy and with age. 30 mm/h may be normal in the elderly. Level raised in most infections, rheumatoid arthritis, myeloma and giant cell arteritis
S	C1 Esterase inhibitor	Plain	5 ml	(See C1 Esterase)	
B	Ethanol	Fluoride-oxalate	2 ml	(See Alcohol)	
P	Ethosuximide	Heparin	5 ml		Usual therapeutic range 40–100 mg/l
F	Fat balance	See Diagnostic Tests for Malabsorption p 221			Approximate reference value is less than 18 mmol/24h (5g/24h)

System	Test	Container	Volume	Reference value	Remarks
S	Ferritin	Plain	5 ml	10–200 μg/l	1 μg/l of ferritin corresponds to 8 mg of storage iron (Adult body iron normally about 4 g)
S	α₁-Fetoprotein (AFP)	Plain	3 ml	2–16 μg/l (non pregnant adults) maternal levels 30–500 μg/l (at 17 weeks 20–100 μg/l)	Increased in intrauterine death and anencephaly. Levels of over 100 μg/l associated with carcinoma. Of no value for early detection. Used for follow up of teratomatous tumours. Transient increase in liver infections. Lower levels of increase in biliary atresia. *See* Amniotic fluid
P	Fibrinogen	Citrate (Verify with own laboratory)	2 ml	2–4 g/l	Increased in nephrosis, infections and after trauma. Decreased in severe liver damage. *See* Defibrination syndrome
	Fibrocystic disease of pancreas	(*See* Sweat Sodium)			
B	Filariae	Thick and thin films should be made at the appropriate time of day for the microfilariae to be in the peripheral blood			Immunofluorescence test (1 ml serum) is positive in most cases of active filariasis, but false positives do occur
S	Folate	Plain	10 ml	6–40 nmol/l (3–20 μg/l)	*See* Diagnostic Tests for Malabsorption *p* 223 Low levels can be found in nutritional deficiencies and pregnancy

System	Test	Container	Volume	Reference value	Remarks
S	Free T$_4$	Plain	5 ml	See Thyroxine (free T$_4$)	
S	FSH (follicle stimulating hormone)	Plain or Heparin	5 ml	Males 1–10 U/l Females 3–12 U/l	The range varies with the time of the menstrual cycle. No special conditions are required for the test except that if serum cannot be despatched immediately it should be stored at –20°C. It is essential to include clinical details with the request. May help to identify primary or secondary ovarian/testicular failure. Level raised after the menopause (with intact pituitary function)
U	FSH	10 ml 2g/dl boric acid	24 h	Males 2–22 U/24 h	
S	FTI (free thyroxine index)	Plain	5 ml	50–155 (4–12) Check with own laboratory. Varies with methods used	This ratio corrects for the divergence of the T$_4$ and T$_3$ resin uptake in pregnancy and when on oestrogens. Increased in hyperthyroidism, decreased in hypothyroidism. See Thyroid function tests
B	Fungal antibodies	Plain	10 ml		
B	Galactosaemia	Fluoride-oxalate	2 ml	Congenital disorder due to hepatic enzyme deficiency. Infant fails to thrive on milk diet. Show enzyme deficiency in RBC of cord blood. Blood galactose normally less than 5 mg/dl (0.3 mmol/l)	
U	Galactosuria	1/100 of 1% merthiolate			Galactosuria-screen for reducing sugars and confirm by chromatography

System	Test	Container	Volume	Reference value	Remarks
P	Gastrin	Heparin	10 ml	Fasting usually below 100 ng/l (50 pmol/l)	See Gastric function tests p 215
S	GCFT (gonococcal complement fixation test)	Plain	5 ml		May be of value in investigation of monoarthritis
S	Gentamicin	Plain or heparin	5 ml	0.5–8.0 μg/ml (mg/l) (therapeutic range)	Peak levels 1–2 h after administration. Trough levels just before dose
S	Giardiasis	Plain	5 ml		Immunofluorescence test positive (at 1/20) in most cases with malabsorption. Trophozoites can usually be demonstrated in squashed jejunal mucosa preparations. Routine faecal examination may disclose cysts of G. lamblia
S	Glandular fever	Plain Sequestrene	5 ml 2 ml		Sheep blood cells have receptors interacting with the Paul-Bunnell antibody characteristic of glandular fever (infective mononucleosis). Screening tests usually positive at some stage of glandular fever. Atypical mononuclear cells present in the blood film

System	Test	Container	Volume	Reference value	Remarks
S	Globulin (total)	Plain	10 ml	20–35 g/l	*See* Immunoglobulins and Protein (total). Globulin is a term for plasma (or serum) proteins other than albumin. In summary, the α_1-globulins contain α_1-antitrypsin mainly, along with α-lipoproteins. The α_2-globulins contain the haptoglobins and the α_2-macroglobulins. The β-globulins contain transferrin and the β-lipoproteins. The δ-globulins contain the immunoglobulins, anti-haemophilic globulin, prothrombin. If over 50 g/l consider liver disease, myeloma and inflammation
P	Glucagon	Special	5 ml	Below 100 ng/l (fasting and at rest) Verify level with own laboratory.	Only of value in the diagnosis of glucagonoma when the plasma levels may be over 1 000 ng/l. The blood should be collected into a heparin tube containing 0.2 ml Aprotinin (Trasylol) and immediately separated and stored at –20°C
c.s.f.	Glucose	Fluoride-oxalate	0.5–1.0 ml	2.5–4.5 mmol/l (45–80 mg/dl)	*See* Cerebrospinal Fluid *p* 212

System	Test	Container	Volume	Reference value	Remarks
P or B	Glucose (venous)	Fluoride-oxalate	2 ml	Fasting 3.0–5.6 mmol/l (55–100 mg/dl) Conversion factor 0.055 At birth 1.6–4.5 mmol/l	Significant differences in level depending on sample and method. Less than 2.25 mmol/l often associated with hypoglycaemic symptoms. See Diagnostic Tests in Diabetes. (For approximate conversion from SI units to traditional units multiply figure by 18) p 212
U	Glucose	Plain	20 ml	0–1.1 mmol/l (0–0.2 g/dl)	Normally negative to screening tests. See Diagnostic Tests in Diabetes. Use 5 ml/l of 5% aqueous chlorhexidine if preservative required
S	Gluten antibodies	Plain	5 ml		Titres rise if coeliac patient on diet takes gluten
Erys	G6PD (glucose-6-phosphate dehydrogenase 1.1.1.49)	Sequestrene and citrate	5 ml	120–240 u/10^{12} Erys	Deficiency associated with haemolytic anaemia, e.g. following ingestion of primaquine or fava bean. Level can be normal just after an episode of haemolysis. (Other enzyme defects have been described)
S	Glutamyl transferase (GMT 2.3.2.2. δ-glutamyl transpeptidase, δ GT)	Plain	5 ml	2–39 U/l (3OU/l upper limit in females)	Levels parallel alkaline phosphatase in cholestasis but often rise earlier. Not altered by bone disease. Of particular value in alcoholic cirrhosis. Raised activity in some kidney diseases

System	Test	Container	Volume	Reference value	Remarks
S	Glutethimide	Plain	5 ml	(See Doriden)	
	Gonadotrophins	(See HCG, FSH, LH)			
B	Grouping (ABO & Rh)	Plain	10 ml		
	Growth hormone	Plain	5 ml		See Adrenal pituitary function tests p 209
B	pH	Heparin		7.36–7.42	See Blood pH and Gas determinations
B	Haematocrit	Sequestrene	2 ml		See PCV
B	Haemochromatosis	(See Iron and Iron-binding capacity)			
B	Haemoglobin (Hb)	Sequestrene	2–4 ml	Adult male 13–18 g/dl (8.0–11.2 mmol/l) Newborn 14–20 g/dl Female 11.5–16.5 g/dl 1-year-old child 11–12 g/dl	Measure of oxygen carrying power of the blood. Reduced in anaemia and after haemorrhage. Increased in polycythaemia
B	Haemoglobin A_1C	Sequestrene	2 ml	3–7%	See Diabetes in Diagnostic Tests section
B	Haemoglobin S	(See Sickle cells)			
F	Haemoglobin	(See Occult blood)			
P	Haemoglobin	Heparin	5 ml	0.5–5.0 mg/dl	Measure of intravascular haemolysis. Sometimes increased after exercise

System	Test	Container	Volume	Reference value	Remarks
B	Haemoglobinopathies	Sequestrene	5 ml		Genetic variants of haemoglobin. Normally 2% of total Hb is HbA$_2$; HbF is seldom present after 1 year. Manifest as a type of haemolytic anaemia. Detected by electrophoresis of a red cell haemolysate. *See* Reticulocytes, Methaemoglobin, Sickle cells, Osmotic fragility and Red cell inclusion bodies. Establish ethnic group of patient
S	Haptoglobins	Plain	5 ml	20-125 μmol/l (0.3-2.0 g/l)	An α_2 globulin. Reduced in haemolytic anaemias. Increased in pregnancy, chronic infection and steroid therapy. Combines with released haemoglobin in red cell destruction
U	Hartnup disease		20 ml		Increased concentration of neutral amino acids. Clinical picture of mental retardation
P or S	HCG (human chorionic gonadotrophin) β subunit	Sequestrene or plain (check which required)	10 ml	Less than 5 U/l (non-pregnant)	Usually less than 1U/l. For detection and follow up of choriocarcinoma and teratoma. Cerebrospinal fluid can be tested when the plasma/c.s.f. ratio of less than 50:1 suggests brain metastases. (The β subunit assay reduces the cross-reaction with LH)
U	HCG (LH also detected)	2g/dl boric acid	10 ml 24 h	Non-pregnant level less than 150 iu/24 h. Maximum over 150000 iu/24 h at 10 weeks	Of value in following up patients with hydatidiform mole and choriocarcinoma and may be of value in missed or threatened abortion and investigations of pituitary and ovarian function. (Quantitative estimation unnecessary for routine pregnancy diagnosis. *See* Pregnancy)

System	Test	Container	Volume	Reference value	Remarks
	Heart disease (ischaemic)	See CK, AST, HBD and Lipoproteins p 220			
S	Hepatitis associated antigen/antibody	Plain	2 ml	See Australia Antigen	
S	HGH (human growth hormone, somatotrophin)	Plain	5 ml	See Adrenal pituitary function tests p 209	
	HPL	(See Placental Lactogen)			
B	Human-leucocyte-antigen HLA 27 (B 27)	1 ml 3.8 g/dl citrate	9 ml		This tissue type has an increased incidence of ankylosing spondylitis. (The tissue type Dw3 has increased frequency in patients with Sjögren's disease, coeliac disease, juvenile onset diabetes and dermatitis herpetiformis)
B	Hydrogen ion			See Blood pH and Gas determinations in the Diagnostic Tests section	
S	Hydroxybutyrate dehydrogenase (HBD)	Plain	5 ml	50–120 U/l	Avoid haemolysis of specimen. An isoenzyme of LDH. After cardiac infarction levels increase to reach a peak at 48–72 h, returning to normal after 7–10 days. The serum activity is also increased in pulmonary embolism and in megaloblastic anaemia. Often normal in liver disease

System	Test	Container	Volume	Reference value	Remarks
U	5-Hydroxyindole acetate (5HIAA)	Add 25 ml glacial acetic acid before collection	24 h	15-75 μmol/24 h (3-14 mg/24 h)	Excretion product of serotonin. Levels may be elevated to 150 mg/24 h with secondary deposits of carcinoid tumours. The patient should not eat bananas during and for 24 h before the test, and should not be on phenothiazines
U	4-Hydroxy-3-methoxy mandelate (HMMA or VMA)	Add 25 ml 6 mol/l HCl before collection	24 h	10-35 μmol/24 h (2-7 mg/24 h) (conversion factor 5.0) 1-5 years 7.5 μmol/24 h	This is a degradation product of catecholamines which is present in excessive amounts in patients with phaeochromocytoma and neuroblastoma type tumours. The elevated levels may be intermittent. Methyldopa, reserpine, nalidixic acid, clofibrate, aspirin and vanilla interfere with the test, depending on the method used. See Catecholamines and Metadrenaline
U	Hydroxyproline		24 h	0.08-0.25 mmol/24 h (10-35 mg/24 h) 6-22 mg/24 h/m² children under 12 months 55-220 mg/24 h/m²	Level often decreased in old age. Increased in conditions of collagen breakdown, e.g. osteitis deformans (Paget's disease of bone). Patient must be on collagen-free diet for 24 h before and during collection; free hydroxyproline (less than 1 mg/24 h) raised if not on diet. Store specimens at -20°C
S	Imipramine	Plain	10 ml		Therapeutic level 0.05-0.6 μg/ml (mg/l) Overdose 1-5 μg/ml

System	Test	Container	Volume	Reference value	Remarks
S	Immunoglobulins				
	IgG			650–1900 mg/dl (75–220 iu/ml)	Level increases at birth but falls again at about 3 months, reaches adult value at about 14 years of age. Increased levels in infections, liver disease, auto-immune disease, myeloma. Polyclonal increase in infections, monoclonal increase frequently implies a malignant process. Decreased levels in hypogammaglobulinaemia (associated with recurrent infections) and lymphoid neoplasia
	IgM	Plain (verify normal range with own laboratory)	5 ml	50–200 mg/dl (65–230 iu/ml)	Increases from very low levels at birth to adult levels at about the age of 7. Increased levels in infections, primary biliary cirrhosis, macroglobulinaemia. Decreased levels in hypogammaglobulinaemias, lymphoid neoplasia
	IgA			90–450 mg/dl (50–275 iu/ml)	Usually absent at birth and increases slowly to reach adult levels at 15 years. Increased levels in infections, intestinal disease, alcoholic cirrhosis. Decreased levels in hypogammaglobulinaemias, lymphoid neoplasia
	IgD			0.5–3.0 mg/dl	A rare IgD myeloma has been described
	IgE			20–300 ng/ml (10–150 iu/ml)	Increased in asthma, eczema, hay fever patients and in worm infestations. Lower levels in children

System	Test	Container	Volume	Reference value	Remarks
S	Insulin	Plain	5 ml	5–30 mu/l (usually undetectable if plasma glucose below 2.2 mmol/l)	Samples should be separated without delay and stored at –20°C. Avoid haemolysis. Blood for glucose must be taken at the same time. Patients should be fasting. *See* Diagnostic Tests For Insulinoma *p* 217
S	Iron	Plain or heparin	10 ml	12–32 μmol/l (60–180 μg/dl)	Take fasting between 09.00 and 10.00 h into iron-free containers. Women tend to have lower levels. Oral iron within 3 days of the test will invalidate the result. Decreased in iron deficiency anaemia and infections. Increased in haemochromatosis
S	Iron-binding capacity (total) (TIBC)	Plain	5 ml	45–72 μmol/l (250–400 μg/dl)	Measurement of unsaturated iron-binding capacity of transferrin plus serum iron already bound. Normally about 30% saturated. TIBC increased but saturation decreased in iron deficiency anaemia. TIBC decreased but saturation increased in chronic inflammatory conditions and often in haemochromatosis. Reduced in nephrosis
S	Islet cell antibodies	Plain	5 ml		Found in many insulin-dependent diabetics. Are indicators of increased risk of developing diabetes mellitus

System	Test	Container	Volume	Reference value	Remarks
S	Isocitrate dehydrogenase (1.1.1.42)	Plain	5 ml	1–6 u/l	Level elevated in liver disease whether obstruction or hepatocellular
	Jaundice			Jaundice is not clinically obvious until the bilirubin level is over 50 μmol/l and at higher levels in artificial light	The usual liver function tests include bilirubin, AST and alkaline phosphatase. Depending on the cause: α_1-antitrypsin, Australia antigen, proteins, GMT, G6PD, haptoglobins, mitochondrial antibodies, prothrombin time and reticulocyte count are other tests which may be required
S	Kanamycin	Plain or Heparin	5 ml		Peak level (1 h after dose) less than 30 mg/l Trough level (just before dose) less than 10 mg/l
S	Ketones (acetoacetate)			80–140 μmol/l (0.8–1.4 mg/dl)	Usually exceeds 2.5 mmol/l in diabetic ketosis
U	Ketosteroids (see Oxosteroids)		24 h		
	Kveim test	(See Sarcoid)			
B	Lactate	Verify procedure with own laboratory		0.4–1.5 mmol/l (3.6–13.5 mg/dl); At rest, arterial level 0.4–0.8 mmol/l	Elevated levels in exercise, tissue hypoxia associated with circulatory failure. Abnormal response to exercise in McArdle's syndrome

System	Test	Container	Volume	Reference value	Remarks
S	Lactate dehydrogenase (LDH, LD 1.1.1.27)	Plain	5 ml	60–250 U/l	Raised levels in cardiac infarction and pulmonary emboli, in megaloblastic and haemolytic anaemia, liver disease and muscle dystrophy. Specimen should not be haemolysed. *See* Hydroxybutyrate dehydrogenase
U	Lactose		5 ml	Negative	Occasionally found in urine of women towards the end of pregnancy and during lactation
	Lactose tolerance test	(*See* Malabsorption *p* 221)			
S	Latex fixation (latex RA)	Plain	5 ml	Negative	A test for antibodies present in rheumatoid disease. More sensitive but less specific for rheumatoid arthritis than the Rose-Waaler test. May only become positive (*i.e.* a significant titre) after some months. Note seropositive and seronegative polyarthritis
B	Lead	Heparin (lead free)	2–5 ml (0.5 ml if capillary sample)	0.5–1.7 μmol/l (10–36 μg/dl)	Adults tolerate higher levels. Rarely have symptoms below 4.9 μmol/l. In children 1.8 μmol/l–3.0 μmol/l indicates excessive exposure to lead, but clinical evidence seldom present until level over 3.0 μmol/l
U	Lead		24 h	0.14–0.40 μmol/24 h (30–80 μg/24 h)	Slightly elevated level in lead poisoning, increases on appropriate treatment, but of little value in monitoring treatment

System	Test	Container	Volume	Reference value	Remarks
S	LE antibodies	Plain	5 ml	Negative	Serum titres of antinuclear factors greater than 1/100 are found in systemic lupus erythematosus. A negative test virtually excludes SLE. Occasionally found in chronic hepatitis and other conditions
B	LE Cells	Bottle containing paper clips or glass beads. Mix	5 ml	Negative	Usually present in preparations from patients with SLE
S	Leptospiral agglutination	Plain	10 ml	Negative	Liver function tests may be of value and sequestrenated blood for leucocyte count
S	Leucine Aminopeptidase (LAS 3.4.11.1)	Plain	5 ml		May be used to monitor feto placental function. No advantage over alkaline phosphatase as a liver function test
B	Leucocytes	Sequestrene	2 ml	Adults 4.0–11.0 x 10^9/l At birth 10–25 x 10^9/l Infants 1 year 6–18 x 10^9/l Children 4–7 6-15 x 10^9/l Children 8–12 4–13 x 10^9/l	Vigorous physical exercise such as a grand mal fit may cause a leucocytosis of up to 30 x 10^9/l, returning to normal after about 5 h. A leucocytosis may also be found in normal pregnancy

System	Test	Container	Volume	Reference value	Remarks
B	Leucocytes (continued)			Differential leucocyte count in adults Neutrophils 2.5-7.5 x 10⁹/l Eosinophils 0.04-0.45 x 10⁹/l Basophils 0-0.1 x 10⁹/l Lymphocytes 1.5-3.5 x 10⁹/l Monocytes 0.2-0.8 x 10⁹/l	At birth the lymphocyte count is about 12 x 10⁹/l falling to 4 x 10⁹/l at 4 years and reaching adult figures at about 10 years. The incidence of infection rises if neutrophil counts are below 1.0 x 10⁹/l due to adverse effects of anti-neoplastic therapy
P	Lignocaine	Heparin	5 ml		Ventricular arrhythmias controlled at 2-5 mg/l
S	Lipase (3.1.1.3)	Plain	5 ml	Check with own laboratory	Raised level in acute pancreatitis. With usual methods it is not as useful a test as amylase
P	Lipids (total)	Plain and sequestrene	10 ml	4.0-10.0 g/l (400-1000 mg/dl)	See Lipoprotein investigations p 220
S	Lithium	Plain	5 ml	Therapeutic range 0.6-1.4 mmol/l (Keep a standard time interval between dose and sampling)	Has a role in the prophylaxis of manic-depression. Signs of toxicity occur at various levels, usually over 2.0 mmol/l. Mainly excreted in the urine. Appears in breast milk
P	Lipoproteins-HDL	Sequestrene	5 ml	1.1-1.5 mmol/l (45-60 mg/dl)	An inverse relation has been found between HDL-cholesterol and coronary heart disease

System	Test	Container	Volume	Reference value	Remarks
S	Liver function tests	Plain	10 ml	*See* Bilirubin (5–17 μmol/l), aspartate amino transferase (5–20 U/l), alkaline phosphatase (20–90 U/l), BSP and Jaundice	
B	Loa loa	*See* Filariae (appear in blood during the day)			
S	LH (luteinising hormone)	Plain or heparin	5 ml	Men 4–20 u/l Verify with own Laboratory Women 5–50 u/l	May be of value in investigation of delayed puberty, cryptorchidism and hypothalamic pituitary dysfunction. *See* Adrenal-pituitary function tests *p* 210
U	LH	10 ml 2g/dl boric acid	24 h	Women 5–75 U/24 h (follicular and luteal phase) 35–160 U/24 h (midcycle) 85–190 U/24 h (postmenopausal) Men 5–45 U/24 h	High levels found in ovarian or testicular failure. Note that there is cross-reaction between LH and HCG
	L/S ratio	(*See* Amniotic fluid)			
S	Lymphogranuloma	Plain	5 ml	Serum for antibodies should be taken before a Frei test is performed	
S	Magnesium	Plain	5 ml	0.6–1.0 mmol/l (1.5–2.5 mg/dl)	Reduced levels in malabsorption and after prolonged i.v. therapy. A magnesium deficiency tetany is described. Raised in renal failure. Avoid haemolysis

System	Test	Container	Volume	Reference value	Remarks
U	Magnesium		24h	2.5–7.5 mmol/24h	
	Malabsorption			See Diagnostic Tests section p 221	
B	Malaria				Thick and thin blood films should be made when first seen and during the pyrexial phase. White cell count, blood culture and blood for Widal test may be of value. Always ascertain where the patient has travelled and note this on the request form (see p 64)
U	Malignant cells			See Special Requirements for Histology Specimens. p 137	
	MCH (red blood cell, mean cell haemoglobin)			27–32 pg (1.7–2.0 fmol)	Decreased in iron deficiency anaemia. (Usually low in thalassaemia carrier states)
B	MCHC (mean cell haemoglobin concentration)	Sequestrene	2 ml	30–35% (30–35 g/dl) (18–22 mmol/l)	Decreased in iron deficiency anaemias
	MCV (mean cell volume)			75–95 fl (75–95 μ^3)	Increased in megaloblastic anaemia and alcoholism and decreased in microcytosis
U	Mercury	Special	24 h	0–50 nmol/l (0–100 μg/24 h)	With severe chronic exposure may have levels over 1 μmol/l. Some normal adults have levels over 250 nmol/l

System	Test	Container	Volume	Reference value	Remarks
U	Metadrenaline—total (normetadrenaline)	Add 25 ml 6 mol/l HCl before collection	24 h	0-7 μmol/24 h (0-1.3 mg/24h)	Most of the catecholamines (pressor amines) are excreted in this form. With a phaeochromocytoma the free amines are greatly increased but only in an active phase. The total metadrenaline and HMMA show less change but are often increased both in active and quiescent phases. Methyldopa interferes with test. See HMMA and Catecholamines
P	Meprobamate	Heparin	10 ml		Therapeutic levels less than 2 mg/dl (20 mg/l). Overdosage levels over 4 mg/dl
S	Methaemalbumin	Plain	5 ml	Negative	Haematin bound to plasma albumin. Indication of intravascular haemolysis. Sometimes seen in pancreatitis
B	Methaemoglobin	Heparin	5 ml	0.5%-3.0% (of Hb) (0.05-0.5 g/dl)	Increased by drugs and in rare inherited defects of enzymes and globin
B	Methanol	Plain	5 ml		Levels of 20mg/dl associated with serious symptoms. Over 80 mg/dl often fatal
S	Mitochondrial antibodies	Plain	5 ml		High titres in most cases of primary biliary cirrhosis
	Mycology	See special requirements for microbiology specimens p 136			
	Myeloma proteins	(See Bence Jones and Immunoglobulins)			

System	Test	Container	Volume	Reference value	Remarks
P	Mysoline	Heparin	5 ml	(See Primidone)	
F	Nitrogen		24 h	70–140 mmol/24 h (1–2 g/24 h)	See Urinary urea
P	Non-protein nitrogen (NPN)	Heparin	5 ml	14–21 mmol/l (20–30 mg/dl)	Includes urea (mainly), uric acid and creatinine
P	Nortriptyline	Heparin	20 ml	(See Amitriptyline)	
S	5′ Nucleotidase (NTP 3.1.3.5)	Plain	5 ml	2–17 U/l	Elevated level in cholestasis. Not raised in bone disease
F	Occult blood	See Occult blood in faeces p 224			
P	Oestradiol (17ß)	Heparin	10 ml	Men less than 200 pmol/l Women (midcycle) 700–1800 pmol/l (follicular) 70–360 pmol/l (luteal) 360–1100 pmol/l (postmenopausal) less than 185 pmol/l	For monitoring ovarian response of women within the reproductive age group and for diagnosis of oestrogen producing tumours
P	Oestriol	Heparin	2 ml	Verify range with own laboratory	Measure of 'fetoplacental function'

System	Test	Container	Volume	Reference value	Remarks
U	Total oestrogens (oestradiol oestrone oestriol)	10 ml of 2g/dl boric acid	24 h	Men 4–40 nmol/24 h Women (non-pregnant) 20–250 nmol/24 h Midcycle 60–300 nmol/24 h Post-menopausal 10–50 nmol/24 h In pregnancy, lowest limit of normal at 30 weeks, 28 μmol/24 h (8 mg/24 h) 40 weeks, 40 μmol/24 h (12 mg/24 h) mean values 30 weeks 90 μmol/24 h (26 mg/24 h) 35 weeks 130 μmol/24 h (37 mg/24 h) 40 weeks 180 μmol/24 h (52 mg/24 h)	Non-pregnancy oestrogens may be of value in the investigation of gynaecomastia and precocious puberty. In obstetric practice used in the assessment of fetoplacental functions. Repeat determinations of greater significance. Test affected by cascara, antibiotics, steroids, diuretics, glucose, barbiturates and phenothiazines
P	Osmolality	Heparin	5 ml	285–300 mosmol/kg (285–300 mmol/kg)	Plasma osmolality is increased in diabetes insipidus and decreased in compulsive water drinking
U	Osmolality		Random or 24 h	40–1400 mosmol/kg (extreme range)	Early morning specimen usually over 600 mosmol/kg. See Kidney function tests p 218

System	Test	Container	Volume	Reference value	Remarks
B	Osmotic fragility	Heparin	5 ml	Normal haemolysis begins in saline 0.5g/dl and is complete at 0.35g/dl. Mean corpuscular fragility 0.4–0.45g/dl of saline.	Red cell fragility increased in many haemolytic anaemias, e.g. spherocytosis. May be decreased in some thalassaemias. Arrange with laboratory; it is a time consuming test and rarely essential
U	Oxalate		24 h	200–450 μmol/24 h (20–40 mg/24 h)	May excrete over 1 mmol/24 h in the rare condition of congenital primary hyperoxaluria
U	17-Oxosteroids (17-ketosteroids)		24 h	Men 17–85 μmol/24 h (5–25 mg/24 h) Women 10–60 μmol/24 h (3–17 mg/24 h) Children 0–50 μmol/24 h (0–15 mg/24 h)	A measure of adrenal cortex and gonadal function. Test affected by digoxin, chlordiazepoxide, chlorpromazine and many antibiotics. See testosterone/oestradiol
U	Total 17-oxogenic steroids (17-ketogenics)		24 h	Men 35–70 μmol/24 h (10–20 mg/24 h) Women 25–60 μmol/24 h (7–15 mg/24 h) Children 5–45 μmol/24 h (1.5–12 mg/24 h)	A measure of cortisol metabolites. Level increased in Cushing's syndrome, decreased in adrenal failure. Test affected if glycosuria or patient on some antibiotics or chlorpromazine. See Cortisol
B	Oxygen (PO$_2$)	Heparin		10.6–13.2 kPa (80–100 mmHg) Conversion factor 0.133	See Blood pH and Gas determinations p 216

System	Test	Container	Volume	Reference value	Remarks
U	11-Oxygenation index	Add 2 drops of 2g/dl boric acid	20 ml	Less than 0.5	Exceeded in forms of congenital adrenal hyperplasia. No preparation required
P	Oxygen saturation	Heparin		Arterial 0.95–0.99 (venous 0.75)	Reduced in cyanosis due to diminished oxygen
P	Paracetamol	Heparin	5 ml	Usual levels are less than 2 mg/dl (20 mg/l or 135 μmol/l). Levels of 20–30 mg/dl (4 h after ingestion) or 10–15 mg/dl(after 12 h) have been followed by fatal hepatic necrosis. Prothrombin Times of value in monitoring liver damage
U	Paraquat		100 ml	If less than 0.1 mg/dl over 48 h after ingestion systemic effects are unlikely	
P	Parathyroid hormone (PTH)	Heparin or plain	10 ml	Less than 1 μg/l (1–34 Amino-terminal less than 120 pg/ml)	Collect at 1000 h. Separate as soon as possible and store at –20°C. Take blood for calcium and albumin at the same time. Level generally raised in primary hyperparathyroidism. Parathyroid venous sampling can be useful in localising the overactive parathyroid gland. A fall in plasma calcium stimulates secretion of PTH which acts on kidney and bone to restore the calcium concentration. *See* dihydroxycholecalciferol

System	Test	Container	Volume	Reference value	Remarks
S	Parietal cell antibodies	Plain	5 ml		Present in most cases of megaloblastic intrinsic factor deficiency (pernicious) anaemia
	Paul Bunnell	Plain	5 ml		See Glandular fever
S	PBI (protein-bound iodine)	Plain	5 ml	300–630 nmol/l (3.8–7.8 µg/dl)	Level raised in hyperthyroidism; reduced in hypothyroidism
B	PCV (packed cell volume or haematocrit)	Sequestrene	2 ml	Men 0.40–0.54 (40–54%) Women 0.35–0.47 Infants 0.45–0.60 Children 1 year 0.35 Children 10 years old 0.37	Decreased when the number or size of red cells is diminished. Increased in polycythaemia. Related to blood volume
U	Pentose	Plain	20 ml		Appear in benign inherited conditions and sometimes after ingestion of fruits
B	pH	Heparin		7.36–7.42	See Blood pH and Gas Determinations p 216
P or S	Phenobarbitone	Heparin or plain	10 ml		Therapeutic levels 1–3 mg/dl (10–30 mg/l) increased if primidone given concurrently
P	Phenylalanine	Heparin	2 ml	60–200 µmol/l (1–3 mg/dl) on normal diet	May have transient neonatal increase. Increased in phenylketonuria to 600–4800 µmol/l (10–80 mg/dl). Heterozygotes detected after phenylalanine load. See PKU
P	Phenytoin	Heparin	5 ml	(See Diphenylhydantoin)	

System	Test	Container	Volume	Reference value	Remarks
S	Phosphatase	Plain	5 ml	See Acid/alkaline phosphatase	
F	Phosphate		3-day	14–28 mmol/24 h (0.4–0.8 g/24 h)	Only used in balance studies
S	Phosphate (inorganic phosphorus)	Plain or heparin	5 ml	Adults 0.8–1.4 mmol/l (2.5–4.5 mg/dl) Children 1.3–2.0 mmol/l (4–6 mg/dl)	Preferably taken from a fasting patient and plasma separated within 2 h. Elevated levels in renal failure, hypoparathyroidism, active gigantism and acromegaly. Reduced in hyperparathyroidism. Levels show diurnal variation
U	Phosphate (inorganic)		24 h	15–50 mmol/24 h (0.5–1.5 g/24 h)	Normally reflects serum level and dietary intake. Increased in hyperparathyroidism
S	Phospholipids	Plain	10 ml	5.0–9.0 mmol/l (150–250 mg/dl) As phosphorus 1.6–3.2 mmol/l (5–10 mg/dl)	See Lipoprotein investigations. p 220
B	PKU (phenylketonuria)				One generally available method (Guthrie) is to collect heel prick blood on special filter paper 5–10 days after birth. Values of 4 mg/dl or over require further investigation. Antibiotics can interfere with the test. See Phenylalanine

System	Test	Container	Volume	Reference value	Remarks
S	Placental lactogen (HPL)	Plain or heparin	5 ml		Used in the assessment of fetoplacental function. Levels are not affected by patient preparation and do not show circadian variation. Levels of less than 5 mg/l (220 nmol/l) after 34th week of pregnancy indicate increased foetal risk. May help with diagnosis in bleeding in early pregnancy. Usually about 0.1 mg/l at 11 weeks and 1.0 mg/l at 20 weeks. Serial samples are of most value
B	Platelets	Sequestrene	2 ml	150–400 x 10⁹/l	Increased after operations and in polycythaemia rubra vera. Thrombocytopenia may be drug-induced. Risk of bleeding considerable below 20 x 10⁹/l
U	Porphobilinogen		24 h	1–10 μmol/24 h (0.2–2.0 mg/24 h)	May be increased to over 500 μmol/24 h in acute intermittent porphyria. Some increase during an acute episode of porphyria variegata and hereditary coproporphyria. Random urine suitable for screening test. Protect from light
Erys	Porphyrins	Heparin	20 ml		Increased in erythropoietic protoporphyria and lead poisoning. Coproporphyrin 1 increased in congenital porphyria. *See* Coproporphyrins and Protoporphyrins
U	Porphyrins (uroporphyrin I & III)		24 h	0–35 nmol/24 h (0–30 μg/24 h)	Increased in congenital porphyria (type 1), symptomatic hepatic porphyria. Smaller increases in acute porphyria, porphyria variegata and hereditary coproporphyria in the acute phases. *See* Coproporphyrins and Protoporphyrins

System	Test	Container	Volume	Reference value	Remarks
P	Potassium	Heparin Separate within 2 h	5 ml	3.6–5.2 mmol/l	Avoid haemolysis. Potassium is mainly intracellular. Slightly higher levels in neonates. Reduced levels with diuretic therapy, hyperaldosteronism, chronic fistulae and diarrhoea. Increased in renal and adrenal failure. Familial periodic paralysis is associated with abnormal potassium levels
U	Potassium		24 h	4–120 mmol/24 h (mean 40 mmol/24 h)	Varies with the dietary intake. Increased by diuretic therapy. Usually decreased in renal failure with oliguria
U	Pregnancy	Plain	20 ml		Early morning specimen preferred. Chlorpromazine administration may give false positives
U	Pregnanediol	Add 10 ml 2 g/dl boric acid	24 h	Men 1.5–4.5 μmol/24 h Women (follicular phase) 0–6 μmol/24 h Women (luteal phase) 6–30 μmol/24h Children 7 μmol/24 h at 7 years of age	Metabolite of progesterone. No special preparation required. May be of value in investigating forms of congenital adrenal hyperplasia and in studying disorders of reproductive function. Multiply μmol/24 h by 0.32 to convert to mg/24 h
U	Pregnanetriol	Add 10 ml 2 g/dl boric acid	24 h	Men 1.2–6.5 μmol/24 h Women (follicular phase) 0.3–5.3 μmol/24 h Women (luteal phase) 2.7–20 μmol/24 h Children 0–4.5 μmol/24 h	May be of value in the diagnosis of certain forms of congenital adrenal hyperplasia and monitoring therapy. Multiply μmol/24 h by 0.336 to convert to mg/24 h

System	Test	Container	Volume	Reference value	Remarks
P	Primidone	Heparin	5 ml		Therapeutic level 2–10 mg/l. It is customary to also measure phenobarbitone, a metabolite
P	Procainamide	Heparin	5 ml		Therapeutic range 4–8 mg/l
P	Progesterone	Heparin	10 ml	0.3–2.0 nmol/l Rising to 60.0 nmol/l during the luteal phase of the menstrual cycle	No special preparation required. Absence of a rise suggests an anovulatory cycle; a level of over 10 nmol/l indicates probable ovulation. Increased in pregnancy
S	Prolactin	Plain	5 ml	Less than 480 mU/l	No special preparation required. May be of value in investigating pituitary tumours and following up hypophysectomy patients. Hyperprolactinaemia is associated with amenorrhoea and infertility in females and, less commonly, impotence in males. Drugs inducing hyperprolactinaemia include metaclopramide, haloperidol, tricyclics and methyl dopa.
	Prostatic acid phosphatase	(See Acid phosphatase)			
c.s.f.	Protein			0.1–0.45 g/l (10–45 mg/dl)	See Cerebrospinal fluid p 211
S	Protein (total)	Plain	10 ml	62–82 g/l	Level alters with recumbency and venous stasis. See Albumin and Globulin

System	Test	Container	Volume	Reference value	Remarks
U	Protein		24 h	0.01–0.1 g/24 h (10–100 mg/24 h)	Increased in nephrosis, in urinary infections, usually in myeloma and, except for the early morning specimen, in orthostatic proteinuria
S	Protein inhibitor system (Pi)	See α_1 antitrypsin			
P	Prothrombin time	Citrate	Measured amount. verify volume of blood required with own laboratory	Control 11–14 seconds	See Clotting deficiency tests. Check the anticoagulant has not leaked from the container before use
Erys	Protoporphyrins	Heparin	20 ml	70–900 nmol/l (4–52 µg/dl packed erythrocytes)	Increased in congenital porphyria, erythropoietic protoporphyria and lead poisoning
F	Protoporphyrins	Suitable specimen		0–130 nmol/g (0–75 µg/g dry weight)	Increased in porphyria variegata and erythropoietic protoporphyria
	Psittacosis	Paired sera and sputum			
	PTH (See Parathyroid hormone)				
	Puerperal fever	Send high vaginal swab and urine for culture			

System	Test	Container	Volume	Reference value	Remarks
B	Pyruvate	2 ml into 10 ml of 10g/dl trichloroacetic acid (Check with own lab)		45–80 μmol/l (0.4–0.7 mg/dl) fasting and at rest	Increased in vitamin B_1 (thiamine) deficiency. Pyruvate-glucose metabolism test may be advisable
	Q Fever				Blood culture may be positive for *Coxiella burnetii*. Raised C/F titre phase 2 antibody
P	Quinidine	Heparin (or plain) 5 ml			Usual therapeutic range 3–5 mg/l
B	Red blood cell count	Sequestrene	2 ml	Men 4.5–6.0 x 10^{12}/l Women 4.2–5.5 x 10^{12}/l	Decreased in most anaemias and aplasia Increased in polycythaemia
B	Red cell fragility	Heparin	5 ml		*See* Osmotic fragility
B	Red cell inclusion bodies	Sequestrene	2 ml		Association with haemoglobinopathies. Are denatured Hb and include Heinz bodies and HbH bodies
P	Renin	Heparin	20 ml (may require more)	0.9–4.5 μg/l/h Verify range with own laboratory	May be of value in investigating young hypertensives with possible hyperaldosteronism and renal artery stenosis. This must be arranged with the laboratory and radiology unit beforehand. The patient must be at rest for the first sample and have been standing before the second 30 minutes later. Specimens should be separated immediately after collection and kept frozen at –20°C until assayed

System	Test	Container	Volume	Reference value	Remarks
	Respiratory distress syndrome (*See* Amniotic fluid)				
B	Reticulocytes	Sequestrene	2 ml	0.2–2.0% (10–100 x10⁹/l)	Increased in haemolytic anaemia, after haemorrhage and during treatment of anaemia, especially in the first few weeks of vitamin B_{12} deficiency therapy
	Rheumatic fever (acute rheumatism)	Throat swab for haemolytic streptococci. Serum for ASO, Full blood count and ESR			
S	Rheumatoid factor	Plain	5 ml	Negative	*See* Latex fixation
S	Rose-Waaler	Plain	5 ml	Negative	Test for antibodies against rabbit immunoglobulin and sheep red cells. Positive in 75% of rheumatoid arthritis cases. May be positive in SLE
S	Rubella antibodies	Plain	5 ml	Consult with your local laboratory. Usually a titre of 1/16 or over suggests previous infection. May require paired sera to decide when infection occurred. Specific IgM antibodies may help decision on abortion. Throat swab in viral transport media may be requested	
P	Salicylate	Heparin or Plain	5 ml	Levels of 35 mg/dl (sometimes reported as 350 mg/l or 2.5 mmol/l) may be reached on therapeutic dosage. In adults consider forced alkaline diuresis therapy if over 50 mg/dl. Levels of over 60 mg/dl can be lethal. Note that respiratory alkalosis is followed by metabolic acidosis	

System	Test	Container	Volume	Reference value	Remarks
	Sarcoid				*See* Calcium. Kveim skin test and biopsy may be diagnostic. Lymph node biopsy (and X-ray investigations) sometimes indicated. Serum angiotensin-converting enzyme raised in about 50% of patients
U	Schistosomes			Pooled terminal specimens of urine should be collected over 24 h. A complement-fixation test (1 ml of serum) is positive at a titre of over 1/20 in most patients a few weeks after exposure	
	Seminal fluid	Plain	1.5–5.0 ml	60–150 x 10^6/ml spermatozoa. pH over 7. More than 70% normal forms, at least 60% motile after 4 h. Fructose present. If less than 20 x 10^6/ml repeat on three occasions over 2–3 months because the count varies	
	Sex chromatin	Buccal smear and blood film			
B	Sickle cells	Sequestrene or plain	2 ml	Test all likely cases before any operation. Associated with HbS. *See* haemoglobinopathies	
	SLE	(*See* Antinuclear factor and Anti-DNA)			
	Smallpox			*See* Special requirements for microbiological specimens *p* 136	
S	Smooth muscle antibodies	Plain	5 ml	Increased frequency and titre in patients with infectious mononucleosis and chronic active hepatitis. Found in association with malignant disease but also in normal subjects	

System	Test	Container	Volume	Reference value	Remarks
P	Sodium	Heparin	5 ml	135–145 mmol/l	Reflects changes in body water. Increased in water depletion. Decreased in diarrhoea, vomiting, diabetic coma, steroid deficiency. Hyponatraemia also seen with inappropriate ADH secretion and in congenital adrenal hyperplasia in the newborn
Sweat	Sodium	Arrange with laboratory		Less than 70 mmol/l	See Malabsorption p 223
U	Sodium		24 h	50–200 mmol/24 h	In general reflects dietary intake, except in renal failure and hyperaldosteronism and inappropriate ADH secretion
U	Specific gravity	Plain	50 ml	1016–1022	Range 1001–1035. See Osmolality
	Spina bifida			See α Fetoprotein	
U	Steroids		24 h		See Oxosteroids and Cortisol
B	Sugar (as glucose)	Fluoride oxalate	2 ml	3.0–5.6 mmol/l (fasting)	See Glucose and Diagnostic Tests in Diabetes p 212
U	Sugar		20 ml	Negative to Screening Tests.	See Glucose and Diagnostic Tests in Diabetes
S	Sulphonamides	Plain	10 ml		
	Sweat test	(See Malabsorption in Diagnostic Tests section p 221)			
	Synovial fluid	Plain and citrate			Volume less than 4 ml. Glucose within 0.5 mmol/l of blood level. Polymorphs less than 25% of cells. Abundant mucin. No fibrin

System	Test	Container	Volume	Reference value	Remarks
S	Syphilis	Plain	10 ml		Flocculation tests (*e.g.* VDRL slide test) often used for screening purposes. Consult microbiologist for suspected early lesions. *See also* TPHA
	TB culture	*See* Tuberculosis			
P	Tegretol	Heparin	5 ml	(*See* Carbamazepine)	
P	Testosterone	Heparin	5 ml	Men 6–60 nmol/l Women 2–4 nmol/l Verify with own laboratory	Plasma should be separated immediately into a plastic container. May be of value in investigation of male hypogonadism, precocious and delayed puberty; sudden female hirsutism and the testicular feminisation syndrome
	Thalassaemia	(*See* Haemoglobinopathies)			
P	Theophylline	Heparin	5 ml		Effective levels depend on concomitant therapy. Aim for 10–18 mg/l
	Thiamine	(*See* Pyruvate and transketolase)			
B	Thrombin time	Citrate	2 ml	*See* Clotting deficiency tests	
S	T_3 binding index (T_3 resin uptake)	Plain	5 ml	117–92 (varies with method)	*See* Thyroid function tests. Is not a measure of triiodothyronine

System	Test	Container	Volume	Reference value	Remarks
S	Thyroid antibodies thyroglobulin microsomal	Plain	5 ml		*See* Thyroid function tests *p* 226
S	TBG (thyroxine binding globulin)	Plain	5 ml	10–26 μg/dl 5–30 mg/l Verify with own lab	Increased level in pregnancy and on oestrogen therapy. Decreased in nephrosis. (T_4 also binds to prealbumin)
S	Thyroxine-iodine	Plain	5 ml	3.1–5.9 μg/dl	
S	Thyroxine (T_4) total	Plain	5 ml	50–155 nmol/l (4–12 μg/dl)	*See* Thyroid function tests *p* 224
S	Thyroxine (free T_4)	Plain	5 ml	9–22 pmol/l (7–17 pg/ml)	Free T_4 serum concentrations correlate well with clinical thyroid status. *See* Thyroid function tests
S	TIBC	Plain	5 ml		*See* Iron-binding capacity
B	Tissue typing	Blood should also be taken in a plain bottle for blood grouping			Arrangements for organ transplantation are now centralised. The Tissue Typing Centre is open 24 hours/day. Notify them and send blood as soon as possible. (Check with your centre what samples they prefer)
S	Toxocariasis	Plain	5 ml		An immunofluorescence test is often positive (over 1/80)
S	Toxoplasmosis (dye test)	Plain	5 ml	Less than 1/4	About 40% of the population show evidence of previous infection. 20% have a titre of 1/128 or more. Active toxoplasmosis unlikely with low or non-rising titre

System	Test	Container	Volume	Reference value	Remarks
S	TPHA (*Treponema pallidum* haemagglutinating antibody)	Plain	5 ml	Negative	Antigen specific serological test for syphilis
S	Transaminases	Plain	5 ml	5–20 U/l	*See* Aspartate aminotransferase
S	Transferrin (siderophilin)	Plain	5 ml	1.2–3.0 g/l (120–300 mg/dl)	A β-globulin. Binds iron for transport in the blood. *See* Iron-binding capacity
Erys	Transketolase (2.2.1.2)	Sequestrene	5 ml	35–90 U/l	Decreased in thiamine deficiency
S	Tricyclics	Heparin	20 ml	(*See* Amitriptyline)	
P	Triglyceride (triolein)	Plain or Sequestrene	5 ml	0.3–1.7 mmol/l (25–150 mg/dl)	Take fasting. Exogenous triglyceride incorporated into chylomicrons. Endogenous appears mainly as pre-beta lipoprotein. Increased in type I, IIb, III, IV and V abnormal lipoprotein patterns. *See* Lipoprotein investigations p 220
S	Triiodothyronine (total T_3)	Plain	5 ml	1.2–2.5 nmol/l (0.8–1.7 ng/ml)	No special preparation required except to exclude patients who have recently received radioactive pharmaceuticals. Increased early in hyperthyroidism and alone in T_3 thyrotoxicosis
S	Triiodothyronine (free T_3)	Plain	5 ml	5–10 pmol/l (3.5–6.5 pg/ml)	*See* Thyroid function tests p 226

System	Test	Container	Volume	Reference value	Remarks
S	TSH	Plain	5 ml	0–7 mu/l	No special preparation required. *See* Thyroid function tests *p* 224
Sputa	Tuberculosis	Three early morning specimens			*See* Special requirements for microbiology specimens. Cultures are reported after 6–8 weeks
U	Tuberculosis	Three complete early morning specimens			
S	Urate (uric acid)	Plain	5 ml	Men 0.12–0.42 mmol/l (120–420 μmol/l) (2–7 mg/dl) Conversion factor to μmol/l is 59.5 360 μmol/l (6 mg/dl) is upper limit in women. The lower levels seen in children	Product of purine nucleotide breakdown. Increased in gout, leukaemia, in treatment of myeloproliferative disorders and renal failure. Test affected by aspirin, methyldopa and paracetamol (depending on method). (Total blood urate 1–4 mg/dl)
U	Urate		24 h	3–12 mmol/24 h (0.5–2.0 g/24 h)	Level influenced by purine content of diet. Urates more soluble in alkaline urine
P	Urea	Heparin or plain	5 ml	2.5–6.5 mmol/l (15–40 mg/dl) Conversion factor 0.166	Lower levels in children, pregnancy and liver disease and on low protein diet. Increased in renal failure, dehydration and old age. *See* Kidney function tests. (To convert from SI units to traditional units multiply by 6 for approximate level) *p* 217

System	Test	Container	Volume	Reference value	Remarks
U	Urea	Plain	20 ml or 24 h	250–500 mmol/l (1.5–3.0 g/dl)	Accounts for most of nitrogen loss, which is balanced by diet. Positive balance normal in childhood
F	Urobilinogen		24 h	50–500 µmol/24 h (30–300 mg/24 h)	Increased in haemolytic anaemia. Usually decreased in liver disease and with complete biliary obstruction
U	Urobilinogen				See Bile pigments
U	Uroporphyrins		24 h	0–35 nmol/24 h (0–30 µg/24 h)	See Porphyrins
P	Valproate	Heparin (or plain)	5 ml		Therapeutic level 50–100 mg/l
S	VDRL (Venereal Disease Reference Laboratory)	Plain	5 ml	A flocculation test used as a screening procedure for syphilis. The reagin antibody detected first appears 7 to 40 days after the infection. A small proportion of patients remain seropositive despite adequate treatment. False positive reactions may occur in association with pyrexia, vaccination, autoimmune disease and pregnancy. The test should be either accompanied by other tests for syphilis or any positives verified by treponemal immobilisation tests or TPHA tests	
P	VIP (vasoactive intestinal peptide)	Special	9 ml	Less than 50 pmol/l	Occurs in mucosal endocrine cells of the gut, Levels increased in VIPoma
	Viral infections	Laboratory diagnosis by microscopy, or virus isolation, or serology			

System	Test	Container	Volume	Reference value	Remarks
U	Virology	Sterile plain	20 ml	Send to laboratory for culture as soon as possible	
S	Virus antibodies			Preferably obtain paired sera, one specimen collected as early as possible in the illness and one 2–3 weeks later. *See* Serological tests in microbiology *p* 137	
S	Viscosity	Plain	5 ml	1.54–1.80	Increased in macroglobulinaemia
P	Vitamin A	Heparin	5 ml	0.7–1.7 μmol/l (20–50 μg/dl)	*See* β-Carotene. After administration of 5000 U/kg vitamin A the level rises to 7–21 μmol/l (200–600 μg/dl) within 6 h, if absorption normal. In Vitamin A excess values of over 5.1 μmol/l, are usually found but some adults will normally have higher levels
	Vitamin B_1				*See* Pyruvate
S	Vitamin B_{12}	Plain	5 ml	160–925 ng/l	*See* B_{12}, Folate, and Malabsorption *p* 223
Lks	Vitamin C	Heparin	5 ml		*See* Ascorbate
P	Vitamin C	Heparin	5 ml		*See* Ascorbate
U	Vitamin C				*See* Ascorbate

System	Test	Container	Volume	Reference value	Remarks
S	Vitamin D (cholecalciferol)	Plain	10 ml	Verify range with own laboratory	Serum should be stored at −20°C and the patient should not have had vitamin D administered in the previous 6 months. No special preparation required. Of value in vitamin D deficiency in rickets or osteomalacia and in hypervitaminosis D. See 1,25 dihydroxycholecalciferol
S	Vitamin E (total)	Plain	5 ml	11–55 μmol/l (5–25 μg/ml)	
U	VMA (vanillylmandelic acid)	HCl	24 h	10–35 μmol/24 h (2–7 mg/24 h)	See Hydroxymethoxymandelate
S	Weil Felix (Proteus OX–2, OX–K, OX–19 agglutinins)	Plain	5 ml		Demonstrate fourfold rise in titre between acute and convalescent sera (rickettsial diseases)
B	White cell count	Sequestrene	2 ml		See Leucocytes
S	Widal	Plain	10 ml	O and H titre less than 1/80	Give details of TAB inoculations. Blood culture, urine and faecal examination may be required. Consult the pathologist and the community physician about notification
	Wilson's disease				See Caeruloplasmin and Copper
	Xylose	Fluoride/oxalate	2 ml		See Malabsorption p 222
S	Zinc	Plain	5 ml	13–18 μmol/l (85–120 μg/dl)	Deficiency may be related to growth retardation, and leg ulcers

Note. Laboratories will often require less blood for a test than is stated in the table because an allowance has been made for variation in the haemocrit and method of assay. Capillary blood collections are often indicated in children. For multiple requests on the same specimen proportionately less blood is usually required than for repeated separate tests. *See* p 140.

DIAGNOSTIC TESTS

Some of these procedures require the close co-operation of the nursing, laboratory and medical staff, and the forbearance of the patient. The doctor should make arrangements with adequate notice and prepare a protocol so that the maximum information is obtained in the shortest time with the minimum inconvenience. He is responsible for the safety of his patient (bearing in mind that pregnancy may be a contraindication), he should know whether the patient is taking drugs or foods which might interfere with the test, and if so whether they can be withheld, and he should be on hand during tests lest a reaction develops.

There are many minor variations of these tests to suit local conditions so check with your laboratory if in doubt, and always confirm the doses especially for children. Details of many of the assays involved with advice on suitable containers and the volume of specimen required are given in the preceding Table of Laboratory Investigations. Reference standards for certain hormones change and this can alter the quoted normal range.

ADRENAL-PITUITARY FUNCTION TESTS

Plasma cortisol

Values are low in primary or secondary adrenal failure and high in most cases of Cushing's syndrome. To demonstrate the normal circadian rhythm 5 ml of blood should be taken into a heparin container at 10.00 hours and 23.00 hours. It is preferable to separate the plasma as soon as convenient. (See p 160.)
Normal (no preparation required)
   09.00–10.00 h 200–700 nmol/l (7–25 µg/dl)
   23.00–24.00 h less than half the morning value.
Morning levels (of patients not on steroid therapy) of less than 160 nmol/l (6 µg/dl) suggest adrenocortical insufficiency. Patients with Cushing's syndrome usually fail to show any circadian variation. In stress situations there is a less marked variation and abnormal results may need to be repeated with the patient admitted and at rest. Cortisol tests (plasma fluorogenic corticosteroids) are affected by fusidic acid, spironolactone, oestrogens and mepacrine, but not by steroid administration, except in high dosage. Fluorogenic compounds do not interfere with tests using radioimmunoassay (RIA) techniques but prednisolone therapy can give falsely high results.

In acute adrenal insufficiency do not delay treatment, which could be life-saving. It should be possible to confirm the diagnosis later with the patient under control. If blood is taken for plasma glucose and electrolytes before therapy, an extra heparin specimen sent for cortisol assay will assist in the diagnosis.

Urinary cortisol

The 24 h urinary free cortisol reflects the circulating unbound cortisol levels. It is elevated in Cushing's syndrome. Using RIA methods, if levels are less than 335 nmol/24 h in males (280 nmol/24 h in females) Cushing's syndrome is unlikely.

Dexamethasone suppression test

This may be used in suspected Cushing's syndrome, if the level of plasma cortisol and urinary steroids are not significantly raised and, in diagnosed cases, to help differentiate between tumour and hyperactivity of the adrenals. Patients with Cushing's syndrome, but not those with obesity, should be resistant to suppression of plasma cortisol levels by dexamethasone. Some obese patients, however, show resistance to suppression, but a single dose test can be used for screening. At 22.00 h give 2 mg of dexamethasone orally. At 10.00 h the next day take a specimen of blood for plasma cortisol. If the plasma cortisol level is less than 170 nmol/l (at this dosage dexamethasone does not contribute to the plasma cortisol level) Cushing's syndrome can be excluded.

When the test is abnormal proceed with a high dose suppression test, giving 2 mg of dexamethasone orally every six hours for four days.

A normal response is against the diagnosis of Cushing's syndrome. If the cause of the adrenal hyperactivity is an adrenal tumour the daily 10.00 h plasma cortisol levels frequently show no suppression. In pituitary-dependent Cushing's syndrome (but not ectopic ACTH conditions) the plasma cortisol levels show some suppression, usually falling to some 50 per cent of the pretest level, over five or six days.

Thirty-minute Synacthen test

This measures plasma cortisol before and after stimulation with Synacthen (tetracosactrin, synthetic 1–24 ACTH Ciba). A normal response excludes primary adrenal failure (Addison's disease). It is often of value to take blood for ACTH assay at the same time.

Take 5–10 ml of blood into a heparin bottle at 10.00 h and then give 0.25 mg of Synacthen i.m. Take a second specimen 30 minutes later. The initial cortisol level should be more than 160 nmol/l and the second more than 500 nmol/l and at least 170 nmol/l more than the first specimen. A 24-hour adrenal stimulation test may be more informative (give 1 mg of Depot Synacthen i.m. after an initial blood specimen and take further blood specimens at 1, 4, 6, 8 and 24 h; the cortisol level should rise to over 700 nmol/l at 4 h). The 30-min Synacthen test can be performed on outpatients but they should remain under observation for an hour after injection.

A three-day adrenal stimulation test will help to distinguish between primary hypoadrenalism and hypopituitarism. Measure the plasma cortisol daily while on 1 mg/day of Synacthen Depot for three days. With severe primary adrenal failure there is no significant change in the levels whereas in hypopituitarism there is a slow progressive rise.

Adrenocorticotrophic hormone (ACTH) assay

It is essential that samples are handled correctly. Fifteen to 20 ml of blood should be taken into a plastic syringe, placed in plastic heparinised tubes and immediately centrifuged. The plasma must be stored at $-20°C$. Transported samples must be deep frozen. There are marked circadian changes in ACTH secretion and haemolysis invalidates the results. At the lower range, with present technology, the results are of doubtful validity.

Normal 10.00 hours 10–80 ng/l   23.00 hours 1–10 ng/l

ACTH determinations are of value in helping to establish the aetiology of adrenal failure and in Cushing's syndrome. In primary adrenal failure levels at 10.00 h are usually over 300 ng/l and are low or undetectable in secondary adrenal failure. In Cushing's syndrome undetectable levels suggest adrenal tumour while values over 200 ng/l suggest ectopic ACTH production, often associated with hypokalaemic alkalosis. Assay may also be of value in assessing therapy for patients with Cushing's syndrome or congenital adrenal hyperplasia.

Metyrapone test (Metopirone)

Should not be performed within three days of stimulation tests and the patient should not be on steroids. It assessses the integrity of the hypothalmic-pituitary-adrenal axis (HPA) and the feedback mechanism.

Metyrapone inhibits the production of cortisol which should allow increased production of ACTH and the degree of adrenal stimulation is shown by increased urinary excretion of intermediate metabolites. This description belies the complex mechanisms involved and, as with many dynamic tests, the results are occasionally misleading. It is a useful test to determine the cause of Cushing's syndrome, but the insulin stress test is preferred for anterior pituitary assessment.

Collect a 24-hour urine for total 17-oxogenic steroids (17 OGS) and a plasma ACTH. On the next day give 750 mg of metyrapone orally 4-hourly throughout the 24 hours (for children—10 mg/kg metyrapone

4-hourly). After 4 and 24 hours measure the plasma ACTH and on the day after metyrapone collect a 24-hour urine for 17 OGS.

With a normal response the 17 OGS and ACTH are increased twofold. Most cases of pituitary dependent adrenal hyperplasia (Cushing's disease) will show an exaggerated response, patients with other causes of Cushing's syndrome, such as adrenal tumours or the ectopic ACTH syndrome, usually show no response.

Steroid insulin stress test

This test assesses the integrity of the HPA axis and its response to hypoglycaemic stress. It is contraindicated in patients with heart disease, epilepsy or on a restricted diet. The patient should be fasting, at rest, and under constant medical surveillance, with glucose available for i.v. administration if required.

Take blood for glucose and cortisol (and other hormone assays, as indicated). If the blood glucose is below 2.7 mmol/l (50 mg/dl) there is a risk of severe hypoglycaemia. Otherwise give soluble insulin i.v. 0.15 units/kg body weight. The syringe should be 'rinsed' with the venous blood. In children, or if the fasting blood glucose is low, it may be advisable to reduce the dose to 0.05 units of soluble insulin/kg. This small quantity of insulin is administered as a diluted solution of soluble insulin. It is best prepared by the hospital pharmacy.

Take blood for glucose at 15-minute intervals for 1 hour and then at 90 and 120 minutes and for plasma cortisol at 30-minute intervals for 2 hours. An indwelling venous cannula is advisable.

The glucose level in one specimen must be reduced to 2.2 mmol/l (40 mg/dl) or lower and the patient should sweat. Immediately the test is finished, give the patient a carbohydrate meal. In a normal person the plasma cortisol value rises by 200–900 nmol/l (7–30 μg/dl). Failure to show such a rise in any of the post-insulin specimens suggests a defect in the HPA axis.

A steroid insulin stress test may be carried out separately or easily combined with other assays to determine the full profile of anterior pituitary reserve. After collecting the basal samples for TSH, ACTH, hGH, gonadotrophins (LH/FSH) and prolactin, the insulin is given, followed immediately by synthetic TRH (*see p* 226) and synthetic LH/FSH-RH (100 μg i.v.). Blood samples for TSH and LH/FSH assay are taken at 20 and 60 minutes, prolactin at 40 minutes, ACTH and hGH at 30-minute intervals for 2 hours as above. Additional testing may be indicated.

A steroid insulin stress test, or some combination, is a good assessment of anterior pituitary function, but is unreliable if the patient has had steroids within the previous 48 hours.

A low plasma cortisol value which fails to respond to hypoglycaemia does not distinguish between primary adrenal failure and anterior hypopituitarism, although patients with Addison's disease are usually more distressed.

Baseline prolactin values give a reliable index of secretion. A normal response to hypoglycaemia or TRH is a rise to over 800 mU/l.

The combination of low plasma testosterone in males (or oestradiol in females) with low LH/FSH suggests pituitary failure. In primary gonadal failure LH/FSH levels are raised. Use of the releasing hormones (RH) allows a separation of pituitary and hypothalamic causes, but occasionally a patient with hypopituitarism requires repeated stimulation.

Human growth hormone (HGH or hGH) assay

Useful in assessment of hypothalamic/pituitary function, particularly in the diagnosis of hypopituitarism, shortness of stature, gigantism and acromegaly. Five millilitres of blood in a plain container required.

Normal adults (fasting and at rest):

       males   Less than $5 \text{ mU/l}(\mu g/l)$

       females   Less than $10 \text{ mU/l}(\mu g/l)$

In cases of suspected pituitary dwarfism if the basal level of hGH is raised this in itself proves that the pituitary is able to secrete an adequate amount of hGH, otherwise single fasting levels are of limited value.

The basal fasting hGH is usually less than 10 mU/l but this level is physiologically raised in pregnancy and there is a marked circadian rhythm with high levels in sleep and is a result of any stress. It is, therefore, advisable that hGH assay is combined with some form of suppression or stimulation test. Exercise may provide sufficient stimulation but an insulin stress test is more reliable.

Growth hormone insulin stress stimulation test

Proceed as for a steroid insulin stress test but take blood for hGH assay as well as cortisol, using an indwelling venous cannula washed through with saline (and heparin, if necessary).

Basal hGH levels rise three- to five-fold on stimulation. Any result above 20 $\mu g/l$ is usually considered an adequate response and below 5 $\mu g/l$ pituitary deficiency is indicated.

Growth hormone oral glucose tolerance suppression test

The routine glucose tolerance test (*see p* 213) is performed, but with blood samples also taken for hGH assay, preferably using an indwelling venous cannula. Most normal patients respond by suppression with at least one hGH level of less than 2 μg/l, whereas most cases of gigantism or acromegaly fail to suppress and may show a rise in hGH.

Glucagon test
Inject glucagon 1 mg (adults) or 0.5 mg (children) subcutaneously. Take blood for hGH assay at 0, 60, 90, 120, 180 and 240 min. The level should rise to more than 20 μg/l. This test is sometimes used as an alternative stimulation test. Its place is not satisfactorily established and it requires attendance for a longer period than an insulin stress test.

Luteinising hormone stimulation test
This may be indicated in cases with low serum FSH values to assess pituitary reserve and for infertility investigations. The reporting laboratory should comment on the results and may suggest a protocol. One regime is to give clomiphene 50 mg twice daily for five days. In females contraceptive advice should be given if necessary. In males continue for a total of seven days. Obtain 3 ml serum for LH assay beforehand and on alternate days during clomiphene administration.

The serum LH level should be at least double by day five. An ovulatory response to clomiphene suggests that control of LH/FSH secretion is intact. Confirm by measuring plasma progesterone one week after probable ovulation.

Water deprivation test
The measurement of plasma vasopressin concentration (usually 1–10 pg/ml) is not easily available and tests of posterior pituitary function depend upon osmolality variations under conditions designed to alter vasopressin secretion.

The water deprivation test is used for the diagnosis of diabetes insipidus. It is important to exclude other causes of polyuria such as diabetes mellitus, renal failure and administration of drugs, *e.g.* lithium and diuretics. It is essential that the patients do not become dehydrated and alternatively that they do not drink surreptitiously during the test.

The patient is allowed fluids up to 08.30 h. From then onwards until the test is stopped no fluids are allowed. The patient should not smoke. The test is carried out under close supervision and the patient is weighed hourly. The test is stopped if the patient loses more than 4 per cent of the initial body weight. The bladder is emptied hourly and the urine volume and osmolality measured. The plasma osmolality is also measured hourly. The test is continued for 8 hours but if the urine osmolality reaches 800 mmol/kg it may be terminated.

In a normal test the urine osmolality should reach at least 600 mmol/kg and the plasma osmolality remain within the range 275–300 mmol/kg.

If at the end of 8 h the urine fails to exceed twice the plasma osmolality and the plasma osmolality is over 300 mmol/kg give the patient 40 μg Desmopressin intranasally (or 2μg i.m.). The patient should eat and drink normally at this stage but collect all samples of urine passed over the next 16 h and measure the osmolality.

In the patient with cranial diabetes insipidus (vasopressin deficiency) the urine osmolality will now usually reach 600 mmol/kg and exceed the osmolality after the dehydration part of the test. With nephrogenic diabetes insipidus (failure of the kidney to respond to vasopressin) the urine osmolality remains less than 600 mmol/kg.

CEREBROSPINAL FLUID

The c.s.f is normally clear and colourless. The pressure, with the patient lying on his side, is usually 70–150 mm (0.7–1.5 kPa). A trace of blood from a traumatic tap will increase the cell count and protein level but in fresh fluid the white cells will be proportionate to the red cells, (see 'bloody tap' p 125). Yellowness is usually due to haemorrhage of more than three hours standing, but is sometimes seen with high c.s.f protein levels, in jaundice, melanosarcoma, and as an artefact due to detergent or skin disinfecting fluid.

Cells
In lumbar c.s.f a count of up to 5 mononuclear cells/mm^3 (5 x 10^6/l) is normal. In untreated acute pyogenic meningitis the pressure is increased and the appearance turbid. The cells are increased to hundreds or thousands per mm^3 and are usually polymorphs. In tuberculous meningitis the cells are increased to tens or hundreds per mm^3 and are mainly lymphocytes. Occasionally a virus infection may have a thousand cells per mm^3 but usually about 200/mm^3 all lymphocytes. In some infections, e.g. poliomyelitis, there may be lymphocytes and polymorphs. Cytology of the c.s.f. may be helpful in metastatic tumours and leukaemia.

Protein
The upper level is 0.45 g/l (45 mg/dl). Proteins are often increased with tumours especially acoustic neuromata, but the most marked increase is found in inflammatory conditions. IgM which is usually absent, is often over 0.03 g/l in acute pyogenic meningitis. IgG, normally 0.01–0.06 g/l, is often increased in multiple sclerosis, when an

assessment of the c.s.f/serum, IgG/albumin ratio can be of value. Classically, increased protein with a normal cell count is described in the Guillain-Barré syndrome.

Glucose
The normal range is 2.5–4.5 mmol/l (45–80 mg/dl). Usually the level is about 75 per cent of the blood glucose concentration. In acute pyogenic meningitis it is less than 1.1 mmol/l and may be absent. In tuberculous mehingitis there is an early fall to levels of 1.1–2.2 mmol/l. It is often normal in viral meningitis but a single examination will not always provide a definite diagnosis.

Smears and culture
In pyogenic meningitis and tuberculous meningitis it is sometimes possible to identify the organism directly on a stained smear and in untreated patients to culture the organism.

The meningococcus may be isolated from blood cultures. In virus meningitis culture of the c.s.f. or stool on cell lines may yield a positive result.

Acute and convalescent specimens of serum for antibody investigations can be of value in diagnosis of virus infections. Serological tests for syphilis are usually positive in late neuro-syphilis; cell content is the best indication of activity.

Lumbar puncture is not without risk and if a posterior fossa lesion is suspected, or papilloedema or a bleeding diathesis is present, it should only be performed after consultation. Suspected meningitis is the prime indication.

DIAGNOSTIC TESTS IN DIABETES MELLITUS

Glycosuria is often the first clue to the diagnosis. Probably non-fasting specimens are of most value. The presence of glucose in the urine should never be accepted as proof of diabetes, hyperglycaemia should be demonstrated. In the elderly a raised renal threshold means that many elderly diabetics do not show glycosuria. During pregnancy most women will, at some time, show slight glycosuria, but a glucose load test is probably only indicated if this finding is repeated or if there is a history suggestive of diabetes.

Blood glucose
Normal fasting 3.0-5.6 mmol/l (55-100 mg/dl). Raised levels are found in diabetes mellitus and some cases of Cushing's syndrome, hyperthyroidism and acromegaly and reduced levels in many patients

with Addison's disease, Simmonds's disease and with a tumour of the Islets of Langerhans. (*see pp* 170 *and* 217). For rapid assessment of the blood glucose at the bedside Dextrostix strips are of value for resolving whether coma is hypoglycaemic or hyperglycaemic. These strips have a limited shelf life (check that the colour before use matches 0 on the chart scale). They can be used with a reflectance meter to provide more precise readings.

If the plasma glucose level is consistently over 11 mmol/l there is no need for a routine tolerance test.

Glucose load test screening procedure

The patient should have been on a normal diet but on the day of the test should fast except for water until the test is completed. Two hours after drinking 50 g of glucose a venous specimen is taken for plasma glucose. A result of less than 5.6 mmol/l can be taken as strong evidence against a diagnosis of diabetes. Any patient with a two-hour value of more than 10 mmol/l almost certainly has diabetes and a glucose tolerance test is not necessary. Glucose values between 5.6 and 10 mmol/l warrant further investigation with a glucose tolerance test.

Oral glucose tolerance test

Preparation is as above but the patient should have nothing to eat or drink (except water) from 2200 hours the previous evening. A fasting blood sample is taken. Following ingestion of 50 g of glucose, blood is collected at half-hourly intervals for two hours. Only if the intention is to investigate possible reactive hypoglycaemia is a longer test required. Venous blood glucose seldom rises above 8.4 mmol/l and in healthy subjects under the age of 40 it always returns to below 6 mmol/l within two hours.

If urine samples are taken at one and two hours from the start of the test, examination for glucose may be helpful in renal glycosuria and to draw attention to a raised renal threshold.

Oral glucose tolerance tests are not reproducible and provide no useful information about the severity or the progression of the disease. They should be performed during the morning. Several drugs affect glucose tolerance, for example, thiazides, steroids, nicotinic acid, phenytoin, probenecid and oral contraceptives may produce hyperglycaemia and propranolol, sulphonyl urea, salicylates, phenylbutazone and monoamine oxidase inhibitors may produce hypoglycaemia. These tests are also affected by endocrine disease and operations such as gastrectomy. A lag storage curve has been observed after gastrectomy when the peak glucose level exceeds the renal threshold while the two hour value is within or below the normal limits.

For children give 1.75g of glucose per kg of body weight up to a maximum of 50 g with a minimum of 10 g.

Many patients find glucose sickly but if they vomit a little this is unlikely to invalidate the test. Flavouring of the solution may help to avoid nausea. A proprietary glucose drink such as Lucozade (volume calculated on the glucose content, about 235 ml) is usually found very acceptable.

Cortisone glucose tolerance test

Give 50 mg of cortisone by mouth eight hours before and a further 50 mg two hours before the test. The rest of the test is performed as for the oral glucose tolerance test. An abnormal cortisone glucose tolerance test taken in conjunction with other findings may suggest latent diabetes.

Management of diabetic patients

When information is required to guide therapy, collect blood specimens for glucose analysis three or four times through the day. Testing the urine for glycosuria at the same time may prove of help if urine tests are later used for controlling therapy. In the elderly patient on chlorpropamide (Diabinese) a blood glucose test before breakfast may disclose hypoglycaemia.

Monitoring blood glucose levels provides a means of better control than urine testing especially as in childhood and pregnancy the renal threshold varies. Some patients can be instructed to test their own blood at home using a reflectance meter and Dextrostix.

Glycosylated haemoglobin A_1c concentration is regarded as an index of the degree of blood sugar control over the previous week. (*see* p 171).

TESTS OF GASTRIC FUNCTION

Analysis of gastric contents is often unrewarding. It requires a relatively large investment of time by the doctor and other methods of investigation are far more useful.

Examination may be indicated to determine whether anacidity is present in a patient with macrocytic anaemia and neurological symptoms; to measure the amount of acid produced in a patient with suspected duodenal ulcer; to reveal the characteristic hypersecretory state of the Zollinger-Ellison syndromes, or to determine the completeness of vagotomy.

Pentagastrin test

Weigh the patient. Omit breakfast. At 09.00 hours pass a radio-opaque

Ryle's tube (size 12-16 French) or a Levin tube (14-16 F or 8-9 E), using X-ray screening to position correctly. The patient leans forward and moves to the left and right while the stomach is emptied with a hand syringe. Place all this specimen of gastric juice into a bottle labelled 'fasting juice'. The patient then lies on the left side and spits all saliva into a bowl. Aspirate with a syringe at frequent intervals for the next hour. Place all these specimens into a bottle labelled 'basal collection'. If need be, unblock the tube by injecting air. Give pentagastrin (Peptavlon) (6 μg/kg) subcutaneously. Collect all gastric juice for a further 90 minutes, label 'post stimulation'. Send the separate containers to the laboratory. A more precise measurement is obtained by collecting separate 15-minute samples.

The fasting juice volume should be 20-100 ml. The basal acid output should be 0-5 mmol/h and the maximal acid output, after stimulation, 5-40 mmol/h in men and 2-25 mmol/h in women. Anacidity is defined as a pH greater than 6 in all specimens. In the Zollinger-Ellison syndromes the basal rate of acid output is over 40 per cent of the maximal stimulation rate.

Most patients with Zollinger-Ellison syndromes have a fasting plasma gastrin level of over 500 ng/l compared with a normal of less than 100 ng/l (50 pmol/l) in young adults. Two 10 ml fasting blood samples are required in heparin but no other preparation is necessary. The plasma is separated immediately and deep frozen. A plasma gastrin estimation is only justified when excessive basal gastric acid secretion has been demonstrated. The plasma gastrin level is raised in uraemia, hypercalcaemia and hypochlorhydria where administration of hydrochloric acid reduces the level.

Insulin test
The test should not be performed within six months of vagotomy. Take 2 ml of blood into a fluoride-oxalate tube. Check that the glucose is normal. Then proceed as above, but in place of pentagastrin give 10-15 units of soluble insulin i.v. Collect blood for glucose determination and aspirate gastric contents at 15 minute intervals for the next 90 minutes. The blood glucose level should fall below 2.5 mmol/l. An increase of over 20 mmol/h in acid output probably only occurs if the vagi are intact.

BLOOD pH AND GAS DETERMINATIONS

Blood pH, PaCO$_2$ and PaO$_2$ measurements should be made with the minimum of delay after the specimen is taken.

Capillary blood may be collected into three heparinised capillary tubes from the centre of a large drop produced by a deep skin puncture. The tubes are sealed and the blood and heparin mixed using a magnet device as described by the suppliers.

Alternatively, and essentially for patients with poor peripheral circulation, blood is collected anaerobically by arterial puncture (*p* 96) into a heparinised syringe (*i.e.* the needle and nozzle are filled with heparin solution—5000 iu/ml suitable for i.v. injection—the plunger is rotated gently and any excess heparin expelled to waste through the needle). After taking the sample, without leaving air bubbles in the syringe, the needle is replaced by a sealed butt and the blood and heparin mixed by rolling the syringe between the palms of the hands.

If the blood samples are not tested at the bedside, the sealed syringe, butt downwards, is immersed in an ice and water mixture and sent to the laboratory. Gas analysis is only reliable within a few minutes of taking the specimen unless the sample is cooled to 4°C when there will be no significant change within a period of two hours.

Blood pH 7.36–7.42 (45–35 nmol/l [H$^+$])
Maintenance of blood pH within narrow limits is achieved by a combination of homeostatic mechanisms including blood buffers, respiratory elimination of carbon dioxide and renal excretion of hydrogen ions. In clinical practice the blood pH can vary between extremes of 7.7–6.9 corresponding to hydrogen ion [H$^+$] concentrations of 20–125 nmol/l but any change outside 7.3–7.5 implies severe acidosis or alkalosis. In compensated acidosis and alkalosis the pH remains in the normal range.

Standard bicarbonate 21–26 mmol/l
The bicarbonate system is the single most important buffer quantitatively, but unless it is known whether or not the primary disturbance is respiratory in origin, the plasma bicarbonate alone does not indicate whether acidosis or alkalosis is present. If the nature of the disturbance is obvious then, in non-respiratory disturbances, measurement of bicarbonate may be sufficient. (*see pp* 151 *and* 155).

Blood PaCO$_2$ 4.5–6.1 kPa (34–46 mmHg)
The arterial carbon dioxide tension is increased by hypoventilation (respiratory acidosis) e.g. in emphysema or with narcotic drugs and reduced by hyperventilation (respiratory alkalosis).

Blood PaO$_2$ 10.6–13.2 kPa (80–100 mmHg).
Oxygen tension is reduced by inadequate alveolar ventilation or

circulatory failure and it may be increased by assisted oxygen administration. When there are ventilation and perfusion defects in bronchial asthma a low $PaCO_2$ may coexist with a low PaO_2. Halving the ventilation rate reduces the PaO_2 to about 8.0 kPa. PaO_2 below 5.5 kPa represents severe hypoxaemia.

Blood base excess –2 to +2 mmol/l
A measure of the surplus acid or base in the blood. In metabolic acidosis (*e.g.* renal disease, diabetic ketoacidosis) there is a base deficit and in metabolic alkalosis (*e.g.* vomiting of gastric contents, ingestion of alkali) a base excess.

DIAGNOSTIC TESTS FOR INSULINOMA

Demonstration of inappropriate insulin secretion in the presence of hypoglycaemia (glucose level less than 2.2 mmol/l or 40 mg/dl) is required for the diagnosis of insulinoma. If seen during an episode of hypoglycaemia, check with Dextrostix and take blood for glucose and insulin assay. If not seen in an attack, collect blood on three consecutive mornings after a 15-hour fast and with exercise before the blood is taken. The patient should be kept under observation. Almost all patients with insulinoma will become hypoglycaemic with basal insulin levels above 10 mu/l. Other causes of hypoglycaemia may be diagnosed by monitored starvation and measuring at intervals the plasma glucose, insulin, lactate, cortisol and urinary ketones.

KIDNEY FUNCTION TESTS

Urea is the main waste product of protein metabolism. In kidney disease urea is retained by the body and the blood urea estimation is a useful screening test of renal function. However it does not begin to rise until 50–75 per cent of renal function has been lost and the levels may be elevated in other conditions such as dehydration or lowered in liver disease. Normal range 2.5–6.5 mmol/l (15–40 mg/dl). The level is decreased in pregnancy (*See pp* 161 *and* 201).

Monitoring the plasma creatinine concentration is a reliable indication of glomerular filtration rate, but in early renal disease a clearance test, repeated if necessary, is more informative.

Creatinine clearance test
No special preparation required. The patient should be encouraged to drink a reasonable amount of fluid during the test. Measure the patient's height and weight. Collect a 24-hour urine specimen (mer-

thiolate is a suitable preservative if required) and sometime during the 24 hours collect 10 ml of clotted blood for serum creatinine. An exact 24-hour urine collection is not necessary, but exact timing is essential.

The result is expressed in the terms of a clearance rate, which is calculated by the formula:

$$\frac{\text{Conc. of creatinine in urine}}{\text{Conc. of creatinine in serum}} \times \text{ml of urine passed/min}$$

The normal mean is 100 ml/min (with a range of 80–120 ml/min). During pregnancy creatinine clearance rises, reaching a peak of 150 ml/min in the 32nd week.

Taking the normal adult body surface as 1.73 m², a correction for children may be obtained by the formula

$$\text{Creatinine clearance rate} \times \frac{1.73}{\text{body surface area (m}^2)}$$

the body surface area being calculated from the weight and height, using a nomogram. In the elderly the creatinine clearance is reduced.

Creatinine is a waste product of metabolic origin and the amount produced per day is relatively constant. For most purposes it can be assumed that the renal tubules neither excrete nor reabsorb creatinine so the total quantity of creatinine excreted in the urine approximates to the amount that is passed through the glomeruli into the glomerular filtrate. The results may vary by as much as 10 ml per minute on repeating the test without any significant alteration of renal function.

Proteinuria

Increase in the protein present in the urine is an important indicator of renal disease, especially of pyelonephritis. Proteinuria may be transient, as is seen during pyrexia or postural as in orthostatic proteinuria. Non-selective proteinuria is seen in the nephrotic syndrome. Bence Jones protein is often found in the urine in myeloma and is usually detected by electrophoresis of concentrated urine.

Osmolality

The physicochemical properties of solutions, *e.g.* osmotic pressure or freezing point of the solvent, depend on the number of particles in solution. Equimolar concentrations of similar ionic dissociation exert a similar osmotic pressure. Osmolarity refers to concentration in osmols or milliosmols per litre of solution, and osmolality to osmols or milliosmols per kilogram of solvent. The latter is to be preferred with body fluids.

Osmolality is usually measured in terms of freezing-point depression. The principle components contributing to serum osmotic concentration are sodium, chloride and bicarbonate. Normally ionic components make up 95 per cent, but in uraemia and diabetes mellitus urea and glucose may contribute significantly.

If a random urine osmolality is over 600 mmol/kg or 900 mmol/kg after 12-hour fluid restriction then kidney concentrating function is probably normal (see p 210).

Osmolal concentration is preferred to specific gravity (SG) estimation, and although the measurements are not equivalent, a rough approximation is 400 mmol/kg for an SG of 1010 and 800 mmol/kg for 1020 SG. If SG is used it is necessary to correct for protein or sugar present in the urine. Subtract 0001 from the SG for every 0.25 g/dl of glucose and every 0.4 g/dl of protein.

Ammonium chloride load test

Ingestion of ammonium chloride normally causes secretion of an acid urine, but this expected increased hydrogen ion excretion fails to occur in patients with renal tubular acidosis.

On the day of the test no main meals are allowed but the patient may have a light breakfast and drink fluids.

At 07.00 hours the patient empties the bladder completely and this sample is discarded. The patient is given 7 g ammonium chloride (0.1 g/kg body weight) in water or orange juice to drink over an hour. Additional fluids may be given to help the patient swallow the bitter solution. It is worth persisting with the test even though only half the dose has been taken.

Collect urine at hourly intervals for the next 10 hours, or until the urinary pH of one specimen falls below 5.3. Do not perform if metabolic acidosis or chronic liver disease is present or within three weeks of an operation or infection.

Renal calculi

Renal calculi may be idiopathic or caused by infection (often with urinary tract abnormalities), primary hyperparathyroidism, renal tubular acidosis and cystinuria.

Stones are often formed when either hypercalcaemia or hyperuricaemia is present. In the hypercalcaemia associated with hyperparathyroidism the serum phosphate level is usually low and the alkaline phosphatase level raised, with increased urinary calcium and hydroxyproline and the plasma parathormone (PTH) should be raised. In idiopathic hypercalciuria the blood calcium level is normal but the 24-hour urinary calcium excretion is over 7.5 mmol (300 mg). see pp 154 and 187.

A biochemical screening investigation for patients with renal calculi would include three daily serum calcium levels (5 ml blood in a plain glass container, preferably taken fasting and without a tourniquet), and a phosphate, alkaline phosphatase, urea, urate, total proteins and albumin estimation (10 ml of blood in a plain container), haemoglobin level (2 ml blood in sequestrene) and urinary calcium (24-hour collection). The patient should be on a normal diet. The urine should also be tested for excess cystine and if a 24-hour urinary hydroxyproline is required the patient must be on a collagen free diet (*see p* 174).

Stone analysis should be performed whenever available.

An abnormal total serum calcium level may be due to changes in the plasma proteins. Ionised serum calcium concentration is a better guide than attempting to correct for this effect, but if not available, a simple formula to allow for it is:

Subtract 0.1 mmol/l from serum calcium for every 6 g/l by which albumin is above 40 g/l and vice versa for serum albumin below 40 g/l.

In primary hyperparathyroidism there is little change in the serum calcium after 120 mg hydrocortisone daily for 10 days. In most other hypercalcaemic patients the calcium level will fall by 0.25–1.0 mmol/l.

(Note that in secondary hyperparathyroidism chronic hypocalcaemia stimulates PTH secretion and parathyroid hypertrophy eventually occurs; the commonest cause is renal failure. It is not associated with stone formation). Tertiary hyperparathyroidism is seen with prolonged secondary hyperparathyroidism when autonomous hyperparathyroidism develops.)

LIPOPROTEIN INVESTIGATIONS

To establish a normal range for lipoproteins presents some problems because the plasma lipid concentration changes with age, sex, diet, the population studied, recent illness and even the seasons.

Investigation of the blood lipids is indicated in patients with a personal or family history of atheromatous disease. The patient should be on a conventional diet, fasted for at least 14 hours and be at rest before and during the test. Tests should not be performed within two months of a heart attack or other serious illness. Ten millilitres of blood is taken into plain and sequestrene containers. The serum may be used to determine the triglycerides and cholesterol and the plasma, preferably tested the same day, is used for lipoprotein electrophoresis. Total lipids are of little value (*see pp* 100 *and* 200).

Lipids are stabilised and transported in the plasma by forming complexes with proteins. These lipoproteins can be differentiated on the basis of electrophoretic mobility, particle size and density.

The alpha fraction has a high density (HDL) and is composed mainly of phospholipid and protein.

The beta fraction is of low density (LDL) and contains about 50 per cent cholesterol.

The pre-beta fraction has a very low density (VLDL) and consists of 60 per cent triglyceride. This may be a precursor of the LDL.

The chylomicrons consist almost entirely of triglyceride. They normally appear in the plasma after ingestion of dietary fat, but usually disappear within 16 hours.

There are rare genetic disorders in which there is absence of the normal alpha- or beta-lipoproteins but the lipoprotein abnormalities of medical importance are those in which the pre-beta and beta fractions are increased and the HDL cholesterol concentration is low. These disorders are suggested as coronary heart disease risk factors. The Fredrickson classification, based on electrophoresis, allows differentiation into types of patterns which are associated with disease.

Type I has creamy plasma with a raised triglyceride concentration. It is normally an inherited condition of some rarity and does not predispose to vascular disease.

Type IIa has a clear plasma with a raised cholesterol level. In type IIb both cholesterol and triglycerides are increased. These conditions are commonly secondary to thyroid or liver disease but may also be inherited. There is an association with ischaemic heart disease.

Type III has a turbid plasma with elevation of both cholesterol and triglyceride levels and a broad beta band on electrophoresis. Clinically atheromatous disease and an impaired glucose tolerance are found.

Type IV shows a turbid plasma with triglyceride increase. It may be secondary but is one of the more common inherited lipoprotein disorders. It is associated with vascular disease and impaired glucose tolerance.

Type V is similar to type IV but there is an increase in chylomicrons.

Other classifications have been described. Type IIb and IV are sometimes grouped together and a simplified arrangement is to suggest; group 1 (essentially Fredrickson type IIa), group 2 (types III, IV and V), group 3 (I) and group 4 (IIb).

MALABSORPTION

Fat content of stools

Before specimens are sent for a faecal fat examination the presence of pathogens must be excluded. Examination of liquid stools is of doubtful value.

The patient should be on a normal diet without laxatives and the test should not be performed within a week of a barium meal. A normal diet should contain between 50–100 g of fat a day (1 oz butter contains 24 g fat and 1 pint of milk contains 20 g fat).

Obtain faecal fat containers from the laboratory. Note the time and date and start the first 24-hour collection. In obvious malabsorption or intestinal hurry sufficient stool will be passed in 24 hours to provide a representative sample. Otherwise continue the collection for a total of five days. Note on the request form the time and date when the last motion was passed.

If the average total wet stool weight is less than 70 g daily then steatorrhoea is unlikely, but the important measurement is the total amount of fat. In the normal adult not more than 18 mmol (5 g) of fat per day should be excreted, the percentage fat content should be 5–15 per cent and the dry weight of stool should be 10–30 g a day.

In malabsorption the dry weight of stool is greatly increased, the percentage of fat is usually over 25 per cent and over 24 mmol (7 g) a day. In infants the fat content is largely related to the milk in the diet. A breast-fed infant with a faecal fat output of more than 7 mmol (2 g) a day probably has malabsorption, but any child excreting more than 14 mmol (4 g) of fat a day almost certainly has malabsorption. With a low-residue diet the percentage fat content may be increased but the dry weight of stool and the output of fat in grams is normal. With intestinal hurry, although the dry weight of stool may be increased and there may be a slight increase in the output of fat, the percentage of fat is normal on a normal diet.

Xylose absorption test

This is a test for upper small bowel absorption. It is normal in pancreatic disease.

The patient fasts from the previous night. At 08.00 hours on the morning of the test he empties the bladder, discarding this specimen, and takes 5 g D-xylose in 150 ml of water, followed by 200 ml of water. All urine passed during the next five hours is collected at the end of which time the patient empties the bladder, saving this specimen. The patient may have his normal breakfast an hour after taking the xylose.

Normal subjects excrete 9–14 mmol (1.4–2.1 g) xylose within five hours but in malabsorption 3.5 mmol or less may be excreted. The standard xylose test requires accurate urine collection, sometimes difficult in the young child. A single blood xylose estimation (collected in fluoride/oxalate) one hour after ingestion of a standard 5 g dose of D-xylose should give a value of over 1.3 mmol/l (20 mg/dl). A result of less than 1.3 mmol/l is an indication for small bowel biopsy.

Sweat test

In congenital fibrocystic disease (mucoviscidosis) there is a general abnormality of apocrine secretions. The presence of over 70 mmol/l sodium in the sweat provides strong support for the diagnosis. In young children the levels are usually about 30 mmol/l. The iontophoretic technique is preferably performed by those with experience in dealing with children and learnt by observation.

Lactose tolerance test

Protocol as for oral glucose tolerance test except that lactose (1g/kg) is administered in place of 50 g glucose.

In normal individuals there is an increment of at least 1.1 mmol/l (20 mg/dl) glucose. If the patient fails to show this increment and an oral glucose and galactose tolerance test (25 g of each) is normal, then intestinal lactase deficiency may be presumed, although there are methods for confirming this directly. When milk is in the diet the stool is acidic and contains reducing substances and the patient has diarrhoea. Faeces for sugar chromatography should be frozen if not processed immediately.

The sucrose tolerance test is similar except that sucrose is substituted for lactose. In young children an extra blood sample at 15 minutes is advisable.

Glucose tolerance tests in patients with malabsorption have little diagnostic value. In normal absorption there is a rise of at least 1.1 mmol/l (20 mg/dl) and often 2.2 mmol/l.

Vitamin B$_{12}$

Cobalamin is absorbed in lower small bowel and blood levels may be reduced below 160 ng/l in malabsorption. The Schilling test has been used to assess absorption of cobalamin. After body stores are saturated the excretion of ^{58}Co-cobalamin in the urine is measured following an oral dose both with and without intrinsic factor. Normally 7–22 per cent of the dose is excreted in 24 hours.

Folic acid

Folate deficiency frequently occurs in malabsorption syndromes. The serum folate normal range is 3–20 μg/l.

Intestinal biopsy

Small intestinal biopsy is an essential investigation in the diagnosis of malabsorption due to coeliac disease. The test should, however, be used selectively and only when malabsorption of some degree has been demonstrated. Liaison with the histopathologist is required. (*see also pp* 137 *and* 153).

OCCULT BLOOD IN FAECES

To avoid the inconvenience of a restricted diet the test is first made on faeces collected while the patient is having ordinary food. Should three daily tests be negative no further specimen need be collected. If a specimen gives a positive test for blood the following procedure may be adopted.

If possible stop all drugs. Give the patient a diet free from fish, meat, turnips, bananas and raw vegetables. Tell the patient to avoid any brushing of the gums and to report any nose bleeds. After three days of this regime collect a small portion of the faeces each day for three days. Any occult blood now found is of significance.

No chemical test is entirely satisfactory and isotope methods using ^{51}Cr-labelled red cells are employed when quantitative determination of gastrointestinal bleeding is required.

THYROID FUNCTION TESTS

All patients with suspected thyroid disease should have laboratory tests, but they need to be interpreted with the clinical assessment in mind.

Radioiodine uptake studies have largely been superseded by *in vitro* techniques and do not form part of routine investigations. Thyroid scans are used to assess thyroid nodules in the management of thyroid carcinoma and to estimate thyroid gland size prior to therapy.

The protein-bound iodine test, which had the considerable disadvantage in that it was affected by iodine contamination, is now obsolete and has been replaced by assay of the thyroid hormones. (*See pp* 188 *and* 199.)

Changes in the concentration of plasma proteins that bind thyroid hormones affect the extent to which these hormones are available to the target tissues. It is technically easier to measure the total concentration of the thyroid hormones (bound + free hormone) but the concentration of free thyroid hormones should reflect more accurately the thyroid state of the patient. Most thyroxine (T_4) and tri-iodothyronine is transported bound to proteins, mainly to thyroxine-binding globulin (TBG) and proportionately less to thyroxine-binding pre-albumin and albumin. The amount of free T_4 is inversely proportionate to the concentration of unoccupied TBG binding sites. Thyroxine-binding globulin varies under numerous conditions which do not usually affect the thyroid status of the individual, thus the free hormone is probably the active part. (*see p* 200)

Total serum thyroxine (T$_4$)
Five millilitres of blood in a plain container required. Normal 50–155 nmol/l (4–12 μg/dl).

The level is raised in hyperthyroidism and pregnancy and low in primary or secondary hypothyroidism. Levels are higher in children under 6 years and often in the elderly.

Serum thyroxine levels are not affected by iodides. The measured concentration is altered by protein and thyroxine-binding globulin changes such as with chlorpromazine, 'the pill', phenytoin, pregnancy, salicylates, phenylbutazone, nephrosis and steroids. Most of the serum T$_4$ is protein bound and although the free T$_4$ concentration is normally stable the total T$_4$ will vary directly with the concentration of TBG.

Total serum triiodothyronine (T$_3$).
A 5 ml specimen of clotted blood is sufficient for assay of both T$_3$ and T$_4$. The usual serum concentration is 1.2–2.5 nmol/l, but up to 3.4 nmol/l is found in euthyroid patients by some methods. A free T$_3$ Index can be provided to correct for protein binding changes if a free T$_3$ assay is not available.

Thyroid hormone binding test (T$_3$ resin uptake)
Five millilitres clotted blood required. The results are expressed in different ways depending on the method used.

The test measures available protein-binding sites and enables the total T$_4$ results to be interpreted as to whether changes are due to a binding change or a change in T$_4$ secretion.

Use of this test allows correction for alterations in the TBG concentration. A value derived from the product of the total T$_4$ and the thyroid hormone-binding test is called the free thyroxine index (FTI) and this correlates well with the free T$_4$ value. The normal FTI is 50–155 (or 4–12 if traditional units used) and a normal FTI in the presence of slightly raised T$_4$ suggests that the abnormal value is due to protein binding alteration. (*see p* 167 *and* 198.)

Free T$_4$
Five millilitres clotted blood required. Normal 9.6–22.0 pmol/l (7–17 pg/ml). The free T$_4$ concentration may correlate more closely with the clinical thyroid status than the total thyroid hormone level.

Free T$_3$

Five millilitres clotted blood required. Normal 5.4–10.0 pmol/l (3.5–6.5 pg/ml).

We usually find high values in hyperthyroidism and low in hypothyroidism but it is probably only of value to help in the diagnosis of hyperthyroidism. In T$_3$-toxicosis (which accounts for perhaps 2 per cent of hyperthyroid cases) a high serum T$_3$ value is seen in association with normal T$_4$.

Thyroid-stimulating hormone (TSH)

Five millilitres clotted blood required but note that thyroid hormones and TSH can normally be assayed on a single 5 ml sample of blood. Normal 0–7 mu/l. Thyroid-stimulating hormone is the main regulator of thyroid function in man and probably stimulates all processes of thyroid function. Useful for monitoring therapy to detect preclinical hypothyroidism and in borderline hypothyroidism. Patients with primary hypothyroidism always have levels of more than 10 mu/l and often over 50 mu/l. Patients with secondary hypothyroidism should have low or undetectable TSH levels but many euthyroid individuals have a low serum TSH concentration. The level is affected by steroids, salicylates, thyroid hormones, oestrogens, antithyroid drugs, lithium and previous radiotherapy.

Thyrotrophin-releasing hormone (TRH) test

The patient is given 200 μg of TRH i.v. (this releases TSH and also independently prolactin) and samples for TSH assay are taken just before and at 20 and 60 minutes after the injection. In normal subjects the 20 minute level is higher than the 60 minute value. A normal response confirms the euthyroid state. In hypothyroidism an exaggerated and prolonged response is found with the 60 minute level higher than the 20 minute level. Patients with thyrotoxicosis fail to respond. A positive result rules out hyperthyroidism and failure to respond excludes primary hypothyroidism.

The TRH response can be impaired if the patient is on steroids and in hypopituitary disease. Patients with hypothalamic disease often have a prolonged response.

Thyroid antibodies

Two main systems are described. Those directed against thyroglobulin and those against a microsomal fraction of the thyroid cells. A tanned red cell haemagglutination test (TRC) or a precipitin test is often used to detect thyroglobulin antibodies and a haemagglutination

(MCHA) test for the microsomal antibodies. Complement fixing and immunofluorescence procedures may also be used.

These antibodies are present in high serum dilutions in autoimmune thyroiditis. The TRC or MCHA are positive in 90 per cent of Hashimoto's thyroiditis and are also found in one-third of simple goitres and in cobalamin deficient anaemia.

Precipitins are found in 70 per cent of Hashimoto's thyroiditis but in less than 20 per cent of other thyroid diseases.

A suggested thyroid investigation protocol is:

1. Initially a T_4 and a binding test. If the results agree with the clinical findings no further tests are indicated as a routine.

2. In hypothyroidism a raised TSH will confirm primary hypothyroidism.

3. If the tests are inconclusive a T_3 and possibly a TRH test for suspected hyperthyroidism.

4. If a nodular goitre is present other investigations such as a thyroid scan may be indicated to determine the cause.

5. Autoimmune disease can often be confirmed by thyroid antibody tests.

Other uses of thyroid function tests include screening of neonatal hypothyroidism and, in conjunction with the clinical condition, they can be of value in assessing the effect of treatment for thyroid disorders. In the treatment of hypothyroidism with thyroxine the return to normal levels of serum TSH is probably the best biochemical indication of a satisfactory response.

During carbimazole therapy the serum T_3 and T_4 usually revert to normal levels within 2-3 weeks of commencing adequate therapy. In our present state of knowledge the TRH test cannot be used as a prognostic guide in drug treated patients.

After radio-iodine therapy and following surgical treatment of hyperthyroidism a rising level of serum TSH may be used as a guide to those patients most likely to become hypothyroid in the near future.

Safety first
Whatever test you decide is appropriate always obey the safety rules for the sake of the patient, the staff, your family and yourself. No test is safely finished until you are satisfied that all contaminated material has been properly dealt with and, if possible, placed in a suitable container for eventual autoclaving or incineration.

4

Treatment

PRESCRIBING

You will find the following publications helpful:

Prescriber's Journal. This is sent by the DHSS every two months to all doctors with NHS contracts. Keep the secretary informed of your NHS post and mailing address (Room 713, Hannibal House, Elephant and Castle, London SE1 6TE; tel. 01-703 6300, ext. 3477).

Drug and Therapeutics Bulletin. Published fortnightly by The Consumers Association, 14 Buckingham Street, London WC2N 6DS. Subscription: £9.50 p.a.

Adverse Drug Reaction Bulletin. Published every two months by the Adverse Drug Reaction Research Unit, Shotley Bridge General Hospital, Consett, Co. Durham DH8 0NB, £1.50 annually.

Both these bulletins are sent free to final year medical students, doctors in their preregistration year and junior hospital doctors in the first four years after registration as well as to trainee general practitioners and doctors in the first four years after entering general practice.

The 'General Information' section and 'Notes on Prescribing' of the *British National Formulary, 1974.* Current until the end of 1980 when it will be replaced by a quick reference format published by the BMA and the Pharmaceutical Society.

MIMS (Monthly Index of Medical Specialties), 34 Foubert's Place, London W1A 2HG. This directory of all drugs available on prescription in the UK is sent to senior registrars once in every three or four months. Junior hospital doctors can purchase it for £1.35 per copy but your chief who receives a free copy may pass it on to you.

THE MEDICINES ACT 1968

This Act provides for a comprehensive licensing system covering the manufacture, importation, wholesale dealing in and supply of medicinal products and consolidates many previous provisions. It set up a Medicines Commission to advise the responsible Ministers and directs the production of the British Pharmacopoeia. Another body, the Committee on Safety of Medicines, advises on the safety, efficacy and quality of medicinal products for which licences are sought. Another (unofficial) body, the Medico-pharmaceutical Forum, representing various medical institutions and the pharmaceutical industry, considers problems of mutual interest. A Committee on the Review of Medicines has been set up to undertake a general review of the safety, quality and efficacy of the 36 000 products on the market.

Prescriptions

In hospital these should be written on the appropriate form or card. You are not subject to any central direction about what drugs you may use but are asked to confine your prescribing to preparations in the British Pharmacopoeia (BP), the British Pharmaceutical Codex (BPC) and the British National Formulary (BNF). When many drugs with similar properties exist, *e.g.* diuretics and antihistamines, find out which is preferred by your chief. Don't try on your own initiative to introduce some new drug or compound which you have only read about. You have had no experience of it and your chief may never have heard of it. If you do give a new or rarely used drug always check the information leaflet in the package and if you are still in doubt ring the suppliers or the Drug Information Service which some hospitals maintain (*e.g.* The London Hospital, 01-247 5454). Many hospitals have issued recommendations about preferred preparations. Use English and metric doses and avoid Roman numerals. As it is easier to remember what can be easily spoken try to avoid 'nought point' and prescribe in doses starting with an integer, *e.g.* when a dose is less than 1 g state it in milligrams. Put a child's age after his name on his prescription to emphasise to the pharmacist that the medicine is for a child. Liquid medicines should be prescribed in 5 ml and 10 ml doses. If intermediate amounts are prescribed the pharmacist will make the dose up to these volumes.

Except in cases where you retain responsibility for treatment after discharge, patients should get their medicines through their family doctors. Small hospitals without pharmacies or with restricted services can give out prescriptions on form FP10 (HP) for a retail pharmacist. The letters NP (*nomen proprium*) are printed on the FP10 form and this ensures that the name of the drug will be put on the bottle. If the doctor does not want the name of the drug to be given, NP should be crossed out and initialled. If a prescription is one for which an entry is required in the Schedule 2 register (formerly Dangerous Drugs Register) the name will not be given unless the prescriber initials the letters NP (initialling is not necessary in Scotland).

A tip about tablets
Many patients say they can't remember whether they have taken their tablets or not. To meet this problem with its risk of overdosage it is a good plan to use seven small boxes each labelled with a day of the week. Every Sunday one day's dose is put in each box and so every night it is easy to see whether the day's dose has been taken. A proprietary device, The Pillsure, with same object, carries a week's supply. Calendar packs are available for some drugs. If a patient has to take a drug 'for ever' it is better to say rather that it must be taken until he reaches a certain age, say 86. This leaves him hopeful.

Drug names
Most modern drugs have three names:

1. An official or approved name given (with its pronunciation) by the Medicines Commission.
2. A proprietary name under which the drug was first made by the manufacturer.
3. A chemical name.

Thus the substance acetamidophenol has an approved name paracetamol and several proprietary names, such as Panadol. Manufacturers choose proprietary names that are easily remembered but now avoid a name that implies a specific therapeutic effect, *e.g.* Coramine, as experience showed that the implied claim was sometimes untenable. The advantage of the approved name is that it often indicates the pharmacological group to which it belongs. A drug prescribed by its approved name often costs less than the corresponding proprietary one.

Poisons and scheduled drugs
The Misuse of Drugs Act 1971 and the Misuse of Drugs Regulations 1973 are concerned with the issue of 'controlled drugs'. Morphine and other controlled drugs are requisitioned by Sister or her deputy and are kept on the ward in a locked cupboard used solely for this purpose. They can only be given when a dated written prescription is issued by a registered medical practitioner who must state the dose, form and strength and total quantity (words and figures). Each dose must be noted in the register. The rules about (other) scheduled drugs mostly

concern family doctors. They are obtained on a signed or initialled prescription.

Identification of tablets
Since tablets have sometimes to be identified in an emergency you should know in advance where to find reliable information about what the various drugs look like in tablet and capsule form. Colouring of tablets other than where this is specified is not official and pharmacists generally disapprove of recognising tablets by colour. This is because many different chemical substances are dispensed in the form of tablets of the same colour and a particular substance may be presented by different manufacturers as tablets of different colours. Use the Tablet and Capsule Identification Guide in the *Chemist and Druggist Directory*, 1978. A few tablets have full names impressed on them. Others have distinctive markings. To identify these tablets consult *Imprex* (Index of Imprints Used on Tablets and Capsules) by W.A.L. Collier, 7th edition 1977 (price 80p from Imprex, 19 Earl Street, Cambridge). Certain poisons (cannabis, cocaine, LSD, amphetamines and barbiturates) can be rapidly identified by the Government Chemist Drug Test Scheme (BDH Chemicals) which your laboratory may have.

Unused drugs
If you find or are given tablets when a patient dies you should have them destroyed as their exact label and shelf life may be doubtful. Also you would be obtaining them other than in the proper way. Residues of controlled drugs should be handed to the pharmacist, who must observe special regulations about their disposal.

Doses for children
The various methods of calculating the reduction in dose of a drug for a child are now seldom used in the wards. It is better to stick to drugs whose paediatric dose you know well but *MIMS* should be consulted if need be.

ANALGESIC DRUGS

Mild ones like aspirin and Compound Tablets of Codeine BP (Veganin) should be tried first.

Morphine in doses of 10 to 30 mg by subcutaneous injection is the drug of choice for severe pain.

Cyclimorph 10 (BW & Co.) contains morphine tartrate 10 mg and cyclizine tartrate 50 mg per ml to avert morphine-induced vomiting.

Cyclimorph 15 contains 15 mg morphine tartrate per ml.

Narphen (Phenazocine) 2 mg in 1 ml for injection (for cases where morphine would be dangerous).

DF 118 (dihydrocodeine bitartrate) 30 mg tablets. 1 ml (50 mg) ampoules. *Omnopon* (Roche) (Papaveretum BPC) 20 mg = morphine 10 mg.

Physeptone (Amidone; Methadone). Dose 5 to 10 mg. 30 mg is the upper limit. An analgesic without the sedative effect of morphine. 12 mg has the same effect as morphine 15 mg.

Pethidine. Dose 50 to 150 mg. The usual upper limit is 250 mg. It has an action midway between aspirin and morphine and also spasm-relieving properties in the colon, uterus and ureter. 125 mg has the same effect as morphine 15 mg.

Fortral (Winthrop) (Pentazocine) 30 mg per ml for injection three times a day and 25 mg tablets, one every four hours—a useful analgesic for moderately severe pain.

SEDATIVES

During your term as house physician you will have excellent opportunities of learning at first hand the way to use sedatives. The choice is embarrassingly wide so you will be wise to become really familiar with a small number. As all barbiturates are apt to cause confusion in elderly patients they are best avoided.

Non-barbiturate sedatives

Chloral hydrate. This safe old drug has come back into use. A popular preparation is Tricloryl (triclofos) 1.0 to 2.0 g. For children triclofos syrup 1 ml up to 1 year and 5 ml after 5 years (500 mg in 5 ml).

Mogadon (nitrazepam) 5 to 10 mg. This is a very safe and effective sedative.

Dalmane (flurazepam). 15 to 30 mg. Acts quickly and is similar to Mogadon.

Heminevrin (chlormethiazole) 500 mg tablet, capsule or syrup (10 ml). A very useful drug with minimal hangover effect.

Sedatives for children (*see also p* 82)

Triclofos syrup (*see above*). Vallergan (trimeprazine tartrate) 2 to 4 mg per kg by mouth. For more powerful sedation give Phenergan (promethazine) and Largactil (chlorpromazine) 1 mg per kg of each by injection.

Placebo

A placebo (*placere*, to please) is a preparation, usually but not necessarily pharmacologically inert, which acts by suggestion. It is given merely to satisfy the patient's desire for a medicine. It often works simply because of the patient's susceptibility to the belief that cures are impossible without drug therapy. Neurotic patients accept placebos readily but not so psychotics who often resist them. Sometimes when a patient expects to feel worse the reaction to a placebo is an adverse one and 'side effects' are attributed to the inactive substance. You may use a placebo if, after having made a full investigation without discovering organic disease, you feel that the patient needs this kind of ritual as well as your verbal reassurance that you are trying to help him. But it is wrong to use a placebo simply to suit your own convenience. A favourable response to a placebo proves the need for further study of the patient's psychological difficulties.

UNWANTED REACTIONS TO DRUGS

Note
1. Diagnosis first and no drugs unless definitely indicated.
2. Always take seriously a patient's statement that he is sensitive to a drug.
3. Some patients have their own undisclosed supply of drugs. If you suspect this ask Sister to search the locker.

Unusual effects of drugs may result from overdosage (including relative overdosage in patients with renal and hepatic impairment), intolerance, idiosyncrasy and allergy from previous exposure. In addition there may be indirect consequences of the primary action, *e.g.* when antibiotics alter the gut flora. Side effects are the unavoidable and unwanted actions of drugs. A list of these caused by some common drugs follows.

Antibiotics. Penicillin—urticarial rashes up to three weeks after injection.

Gentamicin—unsteadiness from vestibular damage. Rashes (especially in old folk with renal impairment).

Chloramphenicol—aplastic anaemia. This drug is best reserved for typhoid and meningitis due to *Haemophilius influenzae* and avoided in other conditions.

Wide-spectrum antibiotics—diarrhoea and anal soreness.

Antihistamines. Drowsiness, mouth dryness, dilatation of pupils.

Artane (Benzhexol). Confusion and paranoid state.

Aspirin. (A constituent of many compound tablets.) Urticaria, tinnitus, gastrointestinal bleeding, asthma.

Chlorothiazide. Gout, increased sensitivity to digitalis because of potassium loss. Dysuria (without evidence of infection).

Colchicine. Nausea, vomiting, diarrhoea.

Digitalis. Nausea, diarrhoea, pulsus bigeminus (extra systoles).

Disopyramide (Rhythmodan). Urinary retention.

Hypotensive drugs. Methyldopa (depression); propranolol (cold peripheries. Vivid dreams—fewer with atenolol); labetalol (postural hypotension).

Methyl testosterone. Jaundice.

Morphine. Vomiting and abdominal pain. Depressed respiration, retention of urine.

Phenothiazine drugs. (Chlorpromazine etc.) Jaundice, diarrhoea, photosensitivity, Parkinsonism.

Phenylbutazone. Rashes, oedema, aplastic anaemia.

Salbutamol. Tremor.

Steroids. Hypertension, sodium retention, oedema (moon face) potassium loss and increased sensitivity to digitalis. Osteoporosis (fractures of vertebrae). Diabetes (shows up latent diabetes). Peptic ulcer. Confusion, depression and sometimes excitement (probably only in predisposed patients). Triamcinolone causes loss of weight, muscle wasting and post-prandial flushing.

Thymoleptics (Antidepressants)

Phenelzine (Nardil). Hypotension.

Imipramine (Tofranil). Dryness of mouth, constipation, sinus tachycardia, cardiac dysrhythmias (perhaps fewer with mianserin (Bolvidon)).

Diseased states of most organs can affect the action of many drugs other than those used in their treatment. They are too numerous to mention here but are well reviewed by I. M. James in *Adverse Drug Reaction Bulletin* No. 51 (April) 1975.

CORTICOSTEROIDS

There is no real dosage equivalence between the various corticosteroids because therapeutic potency varies from one patient to another but it is useful to know that the following doses correspond roughly to 25 mg of cortisone: hydrocortisone 20 mg, prednisone 5 mg, prednisolone 5 mg, methylprednisolone 4 mg, triamcinolone 4 mg, dexamethasone 0.75 mg, betamethasone 0.5 mg, paramethasone 2 mg.

In some patients adrenal depression following the use of corticosteroids may last a long time and so all patients taking corticosteroids should carry a card giving details of their dosage. Such a card should be looked for when any seriously ill patient is admitted.

DRUG INTERACTIONS

As well as side effects and symptoms due to overdosage untoward results may be caused by interactions between drugs. These can be alarming as when asystole is caused by giving Verapamil (Cordilox) i.v. followed by a beta-blocker. A full list of interactions is too long to be included here but you should be aware of the possibility and review the prescription chart when puzzling symptoms arise. You would be wise to consult *A Manual of Adverse Drug Reactions* by J.P. Griffin and P.F. D'Arcy, 2nd edition 1979, in the library. You will probably find in the pharmacy one of the small booklets on the subject such as *The Drug Interaction Guide of Abbott Laboratories* and *Safer Prescribing* by Dr Linda Beeley issued by Geigy.

ANTICOAGULANT THERAPY

In some hospitals the laboratory takes this over entirely. In others you will have to take blood and adjust doses yourself.

Heparin. For immediate action give 100 mg (10 000 units) by an indwelling polythene tube and repeat every 6 to 8 hours. Estimate the coagulation time before each injection and aim at a dose which keeps it at 15 to 20 minutes. Overdosage can be quickly reversed by protamine sulphate giving 1 mg for each mg (100 units) of heparin.

Coumarin drugs. These inhibit production of thromboplastin and other stages of thrombin formation. Warfarin sodium is commonly used. The initial dose of 20 to 30 mg should be followed by a daily maintenance dose of 4 to 9 mg depending on prothrombin activity. This is expressed differently in different laboratories. If it is by 'prothrombin activity' you should aim to double it. If heparin has been given initially it should be stopped after 24 hours when warfarin will be starting to act.

Special points to note are:

Send the amount of blood requested by your laboratory in a tube containing a measured amount of citrate.

Warn the patient to report any bleeding or bruising. Give him a Konakion capsule to use if need be. Tell him not to take aspirin, Septrin, Butazolidine or more than one glass of wine (equivalent) since an unpredictable increase in the prothrombin time will result. Do not depress prothrombin activity until 48 hours after operation. Contraindications are liver and kidney disease and haemorrhagic disorders. If treatment is interrupted start again cautiously with small doses. Phenobarbitone and tetracycline stimulate the production of enzymes which destroy anticoagulants ('enzyme inductance') and so make bigger doses of anticoagulant necessary. Renal failure potentiates activity as the drugs are excreted in the urine.

Coumarin overdosage can be corrected by transfusion of fresh blood or phytomenadione (vitamin K_1, Konakion Roche) 10 mg by mouth or injection.

WHICH ANTIBIOTIC?

(For which drug to use in meningitis *see p* 248).

If your hospital has an agreed policy about which antibiotic to use you will, of course, adhere to it.

Bactericidal antibiotics like the penicillins and streptomycin can be used in combination and their effects will be additive. There is some antagonism between them and bacteriostatic substances (sulphonamides) and such combinations should be avoided. When for other reasons you wish to avoid a certain drug make sure that it is not present in any combined tablet you use.

Antibiotics should only be used in treatment when there is clinical or bacteriological evidence of bacterial infection. They should not be used prophylactically except in special cases, *e.g.* to cover tooth extraction in patients with heart valve lesions. They could lead to superinfection with resistant organisms. You will be guided in difficult cases by the microbiologist's recommendations based on his sensitivity tests.

Antibiotics which are potentially ototoxic (streptomycin) or nephrotoxic (gentamicin) should ideally be controlled by monitoring blood levels. Seek advice on which antibiotic to use and if there is renal failure choose one which is eliminated other than by the kidneys.

For which antibiotics to use see the Antibiotics Prescribing Chart.

Penicillin allergy

A person who has become sensitised to penicillin or other substance will show an allergic reaction to a subsequent injection of it. Urticaria, asthma and shock may be followed by unconsciousness and death. The incidence of penicillin allergy varies from 1 per cent in the general population to 10 per cent in the chronic sick. You should always ask about sensitivity and accept the patient's story that he is sensitive. He may have a card or a Medic-Alert bracelet to confirm what he says. In case of doubt use another antibiotic. As it is the penicillanic nucleus which is responsible a sensitive patient will react to all penicillins and even sometimes to those from which protein residues have been removed. Not every rash after penicillin is due to it and since a diagnosis of sensitivity precludes further use of penicillin it should be

ANTIBIOTICS PRESCRIBING CHART.

System	Infection	Commonest organism	Effective antibiotic	Comment
Ear, nose and throat	Tonsillitis	*Strep. pyogenes* Virus	Penicillin i.m.→ pen V (erythromycin if pen-allergic) Antibiotic not indicated	Initial therapy with i.m. penicillin then change to oral penicillin V
	Otitis media	*Strep. pyogenes* *Strep. pneumoniae* *H. influenzae**	Penicillin i.m.→pen V or amoxycillin if under 5 (erythromycin if pen-allergic)	*under age of 5
	Sinusitis	*Strep. pyogenes* *Strep. pneumoniae* *H. influenzae*	Erythromycin or amoxycillin	
Respiratory tract	Exacerbations of chronic bronchitis	*H. influenzae* *Strep. pneumoniae* (iii) cotrimoxazole	(i) Tetracycline or (ii) amoxycillin or	Reserve co-trimoxazole for ill patients or if no response to (i) or (ii).
	Pneumonia (a) previously healthy	*Strep. pneumoniae* *Staph. aureus**	Flucloxacillin (clindamycin if penicillin allergic)	*Especially after viral infections e.g. influenza
	(b) previously unhealthy chest	*Strep. pneumoniae* *Staph. aureus** *H. influenzae*	Flucloxacillin and ampicillin or cotrimoxazole	*Especially after viral infections e.g. influenza

System	Infection	Commonest organism	Effective antibiotic	Comment
Skin and soft tissue	Impetigo	*Strep. pyogenes* *Staph. aureus*	Topical chlortetracycline + oral flucloxacillin if systemic toxicity	
	Erysipelas	*Strep. pyogenes*	Penicillin i.m.→pen V	Initial therapy with i.m. penicillin if possible then change to oral penicillin V
	Cellulitis Wound infection	*Staph. aureus* *Strep. pyogenes*	Flucloxacillin (clindamycin if penicillin allergic)	
Gastro-intestinal	Gastro-enteritis	*Salmonella spp.* Viruses *Campylobacter*	Antibiotic not indicated	Clindamycin may cause pseudomembranous colitis due to a toxin from *C difficile*
	Bacillary dysentery Invasive salmonellosis	*Shigella spp.* *Salmonella spp*	Antibiotic usually not indicated Cotrimoxazole	
	Biliary tract infection	*Esch. coli* *Strep. faecalis* (Anaerobic bacilli)	Amoxycillin, or gentamicin, or a cephalosporin	
Eye	Purulent conjunctivitis	*Staph. aureus*	Chloramphenicol drops	

System	Infection	Commonest organism	Effective antibiotic	Comment
Bone and joint	Osteomyelitis Septic arthritis	*Staph. aureus* (*Strep. pyogenes*) *H. influenzae**	Clindamycin, or flucloxacillin, or fusidic acid (amoxycillin for *H. influenzae*)	Treat acute disease for at least 6 weeks and chronic infection for at least 12 weeks *under age of 5.
Renal tract	Acute pyelonephritis prostatitis	*Esch. coli* *Proteus spp.*	Cotrimoxazole	not in pregnancy
	Lower urinary tract infection	*Esch. coli* or *Proteus spp.*	(i) Sulphonamide (ii) Ampicillin (iii) Cotrimoxazole	Select in order
	Recurrent urinary tract infection	*Esch. coli* *Proteus spp.* *Klebsiella* *Staph. albus*	Ampicillin, or cotrimoxazole, or a cephalosporin	For long-term therapy one tablet co-trim. or 500 mg of ampicillin or cephalexin at night.

Meninges *see p* 000

From A.M. Geddes, *Prescribers' Journal*, vol. 17, no. 5, with permission of HMSO.

made with anxious care especially in children in whom rashes are common but penicillin sensitivity is rare. Treatment should be as described under serum administration (*p* 118).

SULPHONAMIDE DOSAGE

The maximum safe daily dose for an adult is 10 g and for the smallest infant 2 g provided urinary output is adequate (1500 ml a day for an adult). Gantrisin (Sulphafurazole) is effective in doses as small as 6 g daily. The poorly absorbed sulphonamides (phthalyl sulphathiazole) may be given in doses of 20 g a day or more. Co-trimoxazole tablets (Septrin, Wellcome; Bactrim, Roche) are a bactericidal combination of trimethoprim 80 mg and sulphamethoxazole 400 mg. Dose 1 to 2 tablets twice daily. It can be infused.

COST OF DRUGS

You should cultivate an awareness of the cost of the drugs and particularly the antibiotics you prescribe. In many hospitals antibiotics account for half the drug bill and there is reason to believe that they are often prescribed excessively or unnecessarily.

CERTAIN URGENT CONDITIONS

These notes on some common emergencies are provided in the hope that they may help to avoid the feeling of helplessness which may overcome the young house physician when faced with certain situations requiring immediate action.

ACUTE PULMONARY EMBOLISM

This emergency may occur in any patient kept in bed after an operation or for any other reason. When a large embolus blocks the pulmonary artery death from circulatory obstruction quickly follows and there is nothing to be done. When smaller emboli cause pulmonary infarction with pleural pain and haemoptysis or if, without infarction, there is suggestive evidence (fever, gallop rhythm, fall of blood pressure with right ventricular failure or even simply unexplained pyrexia with syncopal attacks) you may save the patient by prompt action. Take an e.c.g. Warnings may have caused you to discuss with your chief what line he would like you to take, *i.e.* anticoagulant or thrombolytic therapy. Give heparin 10 000 units i.v. followed by 40 000 units in 24 hours (preferably by an infusion pump) to get the coagulation time down to 15 to 25 minutes and commence an oral anticoagulant. If there are facilities for the necessary tests your chief may decide instead to use streptokinase (Kabikinase), which activates plasminogen and lyses thrombi. Give Kabikinase 600 000 units i.v. over a period of 30 minutes followed by 100 000 units hourly for 72 to 120 hours. The laboratory will estimate the plasma thrombin time aiming at 20 to 30 seconds. Prevent thrombosis after the end of thrombolytic therapy by giving heparin (after 2 hours) followed by an oral anticoagulant. To discourage allergic reactions the initial dose of Kabikinase should be covered by chlorpheniramine (Piriton) 10 mg and hydrocortisone 100 mg. Kabikinase should not be used unless Cyklokapron (tranexamic acid 10 mg/kg i.v.) the antidote is available since severe haemorrhage occasionally complicates thrombolytic therapy. Streptokinase therapy may go on for 120 hours depending on clinical and radiological evidence (pulmonary arteriography and leg venography) of clearing of the thrombus. It is usual to give an antibiotic also.

ACUTE LEFT VENTRICULAR FAILURE AND PULMONARY OEDEMA

The patient wakes with an irritating cough after two or three hours sleep, and then becomes short of breath so that he has to sit up. He is pale and sweating and brings up frothy sputum which is sometimes blood-tinged. There may be wheezing and this perhaps makes you think it is asthma. The common causes are hypertension, coronary ischaemia and mitral stenosis. Apart from evidence of mitral stenosis the history, the presence of hypertension with an enlarged heart and gallop rhythm and an abnormal e.c.g. make a cardiac cause likely.

Treatment
Prop the patient up (unless he is shocked from cardiac infarction). Give morphine (preferably as Cyclimorph) 4 mg i.v. (slowly) and 6 mg i.m. Start frusemide (Lasix) 20 to 60 mg i.v. Perform 'bloodless venesection' by tourniquets on the (dependent) thighs. Give oxygen in high concentration by MC mask and aminophylline 0.25 g i.v. If unresponsive and part of the picture of a hypertensive crisis consider diazoxide (*p* 243).

If the cause is mitral stenosis and there is rapid atrial fibrillation give digoxin in an initial dose of 1.0 mg orally or i.m. followed by 0.5 mg at six-hourly intervals (total dose 2.0 mg).

ACUTE MYOCARDIAL INFARCTION

Many hospitals now have coronary care units. You should make yourself familiar with the working of yours. Without this facility or any monitoring device you will have to deal with a coronary problem on its merits. The patient may present without much pain but as acute left ventricular failure. Having made the diagnosis and probably confirmed it by e.c.g. give morphine (preferably as Cyclimorph) 10 mg subcutaneously or 3 mg i.v. and watch. Let the patient lie flat but prop him up if there is left ventricular failure. Give 30 per cent oxygen at 10 litres a minute by facial mask. Thrombo-embolic incidents are reduced by subcutaneous calcium heparin 2500 units twice daily. Unless resuscitation for circulatory arrest has been decided against in advance you should be ready to perform it. Dysrhythmias are common. For sinus bradycardia elevate the legs and give atropine 0.6 mg i.v. if the BP is also low. When hypotension persists then dopamine (Inotropin) 5 μg per kg per min by continuous infusion (Tekmar drip controller) may help. Ventricular extrasystoles (particularly the 'R on T' type) are warnings that ventricular fibrillation may not be far off. So have the defibrillator ready.

ACUTE CARDIAC TAMPONADE

This occurs when fluid accumulates rapidly in the pericardial sac. It causes sudden circulatory failure with rapid pulse of small volume, low systolic and pulse pressures and a raised venous pressure. If there is known disease of the pericardium or a pericardial rub the diagnosis is easier. Inspiration causes the pulse volume to fall (paradoxical pulse) and the venous pressure to rise because descent of the diaphragm stretches the pericardium and increases the pressure in it. Heart sounds are muffled and the cardiac impulse cannot be felt. In rapid tamponade the cardiac silhouette is unaltered. Immediate relief is given by paracentesis (p 95) and you might have to do this if death threatened before you could get help. You could act with more confidence if the picture was that of sudden worsening of a known case of pericardial disease.

HYPERTENSIVE CRISIS

Very rapid lowering of blood pressure is rarely needed and should not be undertaken lightly for hypotension itself can be dangerous and blindness may result. The indications are unresponsive left ventricular failure, hypertensive encephalopathy, pre-eclampsia and some cases of subarachnoid haemorrhage. When the indication is a phaeochromocytoma or an overdose of adrenaline give phentolamine (Rogitine) 5 to 10 mg i.v. For other cases the best drug to use is diazoxide (Eudemine) supplied in 20 ml ampoules containing 300 mg. The dose is 5 mg per kg and the best response is obtained when it is injected i.v. as a bolus in 30 seconds or less. If the response is poor another dose should be given more rapidly. The effect lasts three to six hours and sometimes up to a day. (It is also used as a blood-sugar raising agent in hypoglycaemia.)

STATUS ASTHMATICUS

This is severe asthma unresponsive to bronchodilators after 24 hours. The following remedies should be used.

Bronchodilators. Give aminophylline in a loading dose of 5.6 mg per kg body weight slowly over 30 minutes and then 0.9 mg per kg body weight hourly for 3 hours. Alternatively use salbutamol (Ventolin) 200 μg i.v. in 5 minutes. Routes other than i.v. are of no avail in an emergency.

Steroids. These should be used as the first step if the patient has been on a maintenance dose or if they have been used or withdrawn within the past year. Give hydrocortisone hemisuccinate 4 mg per kg body weight i.v. every 3 hours. Oral potassium supplements are advisable.

Oxygen (see p 111).

Beware of sedation if not on IPPV. Valium (diazepam) 10 mg orally or i.v., or dichloralphenazone (Welldorm) 1.3 g (2 tablets) may be used.

Use a mucolytic agent, Airbron (acetylcysteine) 5 ml of a 20 per cent solution by nebuliser. Have a suction pump ready. The use of other methods such as tracheostomy with IPPV and bronchial lavage is for your chief to decide about.

Dehydration. Water and salt depletion rapidly develop exacerbating respiratory distress so give i.v. fluids.

Antibiotics. If bacterial infection is a likely precipitating factor commence Magnapen.

CO_2 narcosis

When the victim of obstructive airways disease becomes accustomed to a high $P\,CO_2$ level oxygen may precipitate coma because it (and narcotics) remove the hypoxic drive. If acute infection has raised the $Pa\,CO_2$ level a regime comprising controlled oxygen (*p* 111), assisted coughing, metabolic care and appropriate antibiotic therapy should be instituted. If there is no improvement your chief may arrange intubation or tracheostomy and IPPV.

INTRACRANIAL HYPERTENSION

Do not do a lumbar puncture if there is a papilloedema (except when subarachnoid haemorrhage is strongly suspected). Ventricular cannulation through a burr hole is the best method of reducing high intracranial pressure but while awaiting this you should give 0.5 to 1.0 litre of mannitol 25 g/dl i.v. Failing this you could improvise by giving magnesium sulphate solution 50 g/dl into the rectum. (A vessel if half filled with Epsom salts will yield a 50 g/dl solution when crystals are dissolved and the vessel topped up with tapwater).

THE 'ACUTE ABDOMEN'

The house physician may expect to be suddenly faced with the 'acute abdomen' in the casualty department but may take the view that nothing like that can happen in his own domain. These comments are provided to help him refute the gibe that the worst place to perforate is in the medical ward. The main pitfall to avoid is to call the surgeon too late.

Many abdominal pains are medical in origin but when they last longer than six hours they are generally caused by a surgical condition. A medical and a surgical cause may coincide. Pneumonia can occur with appendicitis and coronary occlusion with cholecystitis. So do not be lulled by the original diagnostic label but examine the patient afresh, flat in bed and bare from breast to thigh. If he cannot raise himself without using his arms an 'acute abdomen' is likely. Palpate the abdomen with the flat of the warm hand, examining the place complained of last of all. Note any tenderness or rigidity and watch the mobility of the chest wall. If it is fixed or recedes on inspiration peritoneal irritation is suggested. Examine the chest (for pneumonia) as well as the gums and jerks. Lead colic and the gastric crises of tabes are forgotten rarities. Do not ignore the hernial orifices and rarely omit a rectal examination.

If you are still in doubt obtain a surgical opinion via your opposite number. He may find what you have missed but it is better to be humiliated at the bedside early than when it is too late for the patient's life to be saved.

HAEMATEMESIS

A life-threatening sudden haematemesis calls for urgent surgery preceded by transfusion and possibly fibreoptic endoscopy. This may be advisable even if there are known varices since these may not be the cause. If portal hypertension is likely (in 5 per cent of cases only) try

Vasopressin injection BPC (Pitressin) 20 units (1 ml in 100 ml of glucose 5 g/dl i.v. over 10 minutes). Oesophageal tamponade (p 80) may be necessary.

The patient with steady bleeding or recurrent episodes calls for close observation. Raise the foot of the bed. Order an hourly pulse and BP chart. Take blood for grouping and cross-matching (p 120). Give dilute saline by mouth and soon go on to puree foods. If the haemoglobin is 8 g per dl or less start a transfusion. Call the surgeon if the patient is shocked, over 50 or if bleeding recurs. Don't bring him only when the patient is at his last gasp. When bleeding from a peptic ulcer has ceased commence cimetidine (Tagamet) 200 mg 3 times a day and 400 mg at night.

HEPATIC COMA

This will concern the HP when in hepatic cirrhosis already diagnosed it arises from natural progress or is precipitated by diuretic therapy or gastrointestinal haemorrhage. It may occur episodically after a portacaval anastomosis. The principles of treatment are: (1) purgation and protein restriction; (2) intestinal antibiotics (neomycin 1 g 4 hourly by mouth); (3) laevulose (Duphalac) 30 ml each morning; (4) general care of the comatose patient and correction of electrolyte disturbances. Bleeding from oesophageal varices may call for insertion of a Sengstaken-Blakemore tube (p 80).

ACUTE LIVER INJURY

This rare emergency is at present mostly the result of paracetamol overdosage (p 267) but other toxins can cause it. Transfer to an intensive care unit is desirable—possibly the Liver Unit at King's College Hospital, London (tel. 01-274 6222 ext. 2196).

TACHYDYSRRHYTHMIAS

Take an e.c.g.

If the complexes are normal and similar to previous ones the tachycardia probably originates in the AV node or above.

1. Sinus tachycardia
Find and treat the cause (blood loss, fever, pulmonary embolus, pericarditis).

2. Paroxysmal supraventricular tachycardia
The patient may give a history of previous short-lived episodes. Try

carotid sinus massage (*p* 96). If this fails give practolol (Eraldin) 10 to 20 mg by slow i.v. injection. If very rapid or in failure use DC conversion. (Consider the Wolff-Parkinson-White syndrome as a cause of recurrent episodes.)

3. Atrial flutter and fibrillation.
Treat with digoxin unless very ill when DC conversion is necessary.

4. Nodal tachycardias.
Treat as for supraventricular tachycardia.

If the complexes are spread (like those of bundle branch block and ventricular ectopics) and unlike previous ones the tachycardia probably arises in the ventricles. Sometimes SVT is so rapid that the conduction pathways fatigue and complexes are spread (SVT with aberrant conduction).

Ventricular tachycardia
Give an i.v. bolus of lignocaine 100 mg. If no response give procainamide 500 mg i.v. at 100 mg per minute. Check the BP each minute. If the patient is very ill or there is no response to drugs give diazepam (Valium) 10 to 30 mg i.v. and when unconscious give 200 joules DC shock (*p* 275). Continue antiarrhythmic drugs after the patient has reverted to normal rhythm.

Digoxin can cause any dysrrhythmia and the best treatment may be to stop it. Its effect is potentiated by hypokalaemia and acidosis. Tachycardia refractory to drugs may call for pacing and your chief will decide about this.

ARTERIAL OCCLUSION

Arterial embolism is shown by sudden 'pain, pallor and paralysis' of a limb in a patient with mitral stenosis or other source of an embolus. Arterial thrombosis being slower is less likely to cause pain.

Do not delay. Give pethidine 100 to 150 mg subcutaneously (not into the affected limb) for pain, if necessary. Give papaverine 30 to 60 mg i.v. and tolazoline (Priscol) 25 mg i.v. Use whisky or brandy in liberal doses.

All these measures aim at causing dilatation of collaterals. Forbid smoking which might have the opposite effect.

Do not elevate the limb. This would hinder its blood supply. Do not warm the limb but leave it exposed to room temperature. This reduces its oxygen requirements. Put a glove on the opposite hand and a bedsock on the opposite foot and let the patient wear his bed jacket. These measures may release vasoconstriction reflexly. Start anticoagulant therapy (*pp* 148 *and* 235) and notify your senior so that a surgeon may be consulted.

CONVULSIONS IN CHILDREN

To be called to a child having a convulsion is a disconcerting experience. Often by the time you reach him the fit is over. If it is not, all you need do is to prevent him hurting himself. When the jaws are already in spasm you may cause damage by forcing them open but a gag may be used if the airway is obstructed. The parents will be alarmed and it is important to behave in a reassuring way. Let them see that you know what you are about. Prevent them from doing silly things. It is comforting to them to see a cold compress being prepared and even to help you or Sister to put it on the head. In the rare case where fits continue without a return of consciousness (status epilepticus) they must be stopped, for prolonged convulsions are incriminated as a cause of temporal lobe epilepsy. Give diazepam (Valium) 5 to 10 mg by slow i.v. injection or rectally. If this fails thiopentone or an inhaled anaesthetic will be needed (call the anaesthetist). After the fit is over try to find the cause. This varies with the age of the child. In the newborn birth injury is likely. Hypoglycaemia should be looked for because it is easily missed and otherwise disastrous. In the toddler febrile convulsions are common and in the older child epilepsy, intracranial disease (meningitis) and nephritis should be thought of.

About 1 child in 15 has a convulsion and at least one-third of these are simple febrile convulsions. So be reassuring to the parents. The outlook is good if the child is mentally and structurally normal and if the fits are brief, albeit recurrent, complications of a febrile illness ('benign febrile convulsions') as distinct from true epilepsy precipitated by fever.

STATUS EPILEPTICUS IN THE ADULT

Give diazepam (Valium) 0.2 mg per kg i.m. or i.v. repeated in one hour if need be. It can be infused (up to 3 mg per kg in 24 hours) using a Tekmar drip controller until fits cease. In elderly patients the dose should be halved. Chlormethiazole (Heminevrin) 1.2 to 1.6 g in 0.8 per cent solution may be similarly injected. If fits are prolonged look to the electrolytes.

THE EXCITED PATIENT

Grossly increased mental and bodily excitement may occur in many psychiatric disorders. It may also be 'toxic' (delirium) so check carefully for infection and drug overdosage and take appropriate action as necessary. Do not restrain the patient except from injuring himself and others. Give haloperidol (Serenace) 5 mg i.m. or i.v. and repeat six-hourly if need be. Chlorpromazine 200 mg i.m. or slowly i.v. may be given as an alternative. Occasionally more is needed. Hypothermia may result from peripheral vasodilatation induced by chlorpromazine.

Homicidal impulses call for prompt action, *i.e.* compulsory detention (*p* 39) to avoid possible murders. Have an attendant present when you question such a patient and remove potential weapons first. It is better to be sure than sorry.

MENINGITIS—WHICH DRUG TO USE?

Once the question of meningitis has crossed your mind you must do a lumbar puncture. Which drug to use will depend on the c.s.f. findings. Have benzyl penicillin 10000 units in 2 ml of water for injection ready and if the fluid is turbid give it intrathecally but reduce the dose to 1000 to 3000 units for a child. If you are not absolutely certain about sterility put a small millipore filter between the syringe and the needle. Penicillin from a multidose pack (with preservative) must not be used. If the fluid looks clear await further c.s.f. findings for the case is probably one of lymphocytic meningitis.

Polymorphs, raised protein and reduced or absent sugar confirms the diagnosis of pyogenic meningitis. Treatment is by amoxycillin 200 mg per kg per day in divided i.m. doses every four hours and sulphadiazine 1.5 g by mouth every six hours for seven days. If all signs of meningitis have not disappeared in this time repeat the lumbar puncture to see if organisms are still present (this is most unlikely in meningococcal cases).

The results of culture of the first c.s.f. should be available within 24 hours and treatment should be modified accordingly.

Neisseria meningitidis. Continue with sulphadiazine unless the organism is resistant to sulphonamide. Substitute benzyl penicillin 1 mega unit i.m. or i.v. every 4 hours for amoxycillin. Contacts should receive co-trimoxazole (Septrin, Bactrim) 2 tablets three times a day for four days.

Streptomyces pneumoniae. Give benzyl penicillin 1 mega unit i.v. every two hours until a good response is obtained, then 2 mega units i.m. every four hours for a week. Sulphonamide as above. If the patient's condition is unsatisfactory after a week re-examine the c.s.f. and if it is abnormal seek a further opinion. There may be a (surgical) focus of infection. For patients allergic to penicillin cephaloridine (Ceporin) may be tried giving up to 100 mg per kg i.m. per day (maximum 6 g a day for an adult).

Haemophilus influenzae. Give amoxycillin as above. (Sulphonamides are ineffective.)

Other organisms. Treatment is according to organisms and their sensitivities. In neonates and young infants assume a Gram-negative infection and begin treatment with amoxycillin 50 mg i.m. every 8 hours and gentamicin (3 mg per kg 12 hourly up to 2 weeks old and 2 mg/kg 8 hourly from 2 to 12 weeks old). Intrathecal treatment may also be required and expert paediatric and possibly neurosurgical care is necessary.

If the c.s.f. is sterile and shows an increase in protein and lymphocytes but not polymorphs the diagnosis is likely to be viral meningitis, non-paralytic poliomyelitis or tuberculous meningitis. (The last is rare but must be thought of in immigrants. Your chief will decide on the correct treatment.)

Never use a battery of antibiotics. It is rarely justified on scientific grounds. Only if the patient is penicillin sensitive or the organism penicillin resistant should the use of chloramphenicol be considered. Nevertheless your chief may be one of those who prefer to use several antibiotics until the sensitivities are known. In a very sick child some prefer to give them by i.v. drip for the first 48 hours.

FOREIGN BODY IN THE EAR

You may meet this problem in a child in casualty. Instil some liquid paraffin and shake the head with the affected ear undermost. If this is ineffective you will have to arrange for a general anaesthetic. Never use forceps for they will impel a small foreign body inwards and even through the tympanic membrane. Pass a strabismus hook beyond the foreign body (the oval shape of the meatus allows this). The foreign body can then be withdrawn.

FOREIGN BODY IN THE NOSE

Anaesthetise the child. Spray the nose with Solution of Adrenaline Hydrochloride BP (a decongestant). Place the child on his back with a pillow under his shoulders (the 'tonsil position'), so that if the foreign body is pushed further on it will land in the post-nasal space and won't be inhaled. Wear a head mirror and pass a strabismus hook upwards and backwards close to the septum and withdraw the foreign body.

EPISTAXIS

Bleeding from the nose only becomes a job for the doctor when it won't stop. Sometimes this is because of inexpert handling at home. It is best to try simple measures first. In 80 per cent of cases the site of bleeding is the antero-inferior part of the septum (Little's or Kiesselbach's area) where the anastomoses between branches of the internal and external carotid arteries is greatest. So tell the patient to pinch his nose between his thumb and index finger for five minutes. If this fails give a sedative [diazepam (Valium) 5 to 10 mg] and make him sit upright and breathe through his mouth. He must stop swallowing. Give him a bowl to dribble into. Only intravascular clotting will prevent recurrence. So if bleeding goes on make the patient blow out all the (extravascular) clot and find out which side is bleeding. Anaesthetise this side with wool soaked in 4 per cent lignocaine with an equal amount of solution of Adrenaline Hydrochloride BP for two minutes. Using a head mirror with a good source of light and a Thudichum's nasal speculum remove the wool and look for the bleeding point. If seen put in an anterior nasal pack (ribbon gauze packed in several layers from below upwards). Bleeding far back or from above the middle turbinate is a more difficult problem calling for a postnasal pack. To place this correctly is an expert procedure needing good anaesthesia and you should call a senior colleague. He may plug with gauze or use the balloon tampon. A catheter with a terminal lubricated balloon is passed along the floor of the nose. When it reaches the post-nasal wall the balloon is inflated to occlude the choana. A mobile balloon on the catheter is then suitably positioned in the nasal cavity and inflated. If you are forced to improvise then pass a Foley catheter along the nose and inflate its balloon to occlude the choana. Having fixed the anterior end the nose can then be packed with gauze soaked in bismuth iodoform paraffin paste (BIPP). Packs and balloons can be left in place for 48 hours if need be.

THE BLEEDING TOOTH SOCKET

This problem usually presents to the house physician as a call to the casualty department to see a patient who has had a tooth extracted during the previous 24 hours and is still bleeding.

Reassure the patient and, if necessary, give him a sedative. Clear the mouth of loose clots, using cotton wool and isosmotic sodium chloride solution. Verify the site of bleeding. Make a roll of gauze like a cigar and put it across the socket. Tell the patient to bite on this. A bandage may be used to keep the jaws together. After 20 minutes remove the gauze gently. This is usually all that is necessary as the bleeding was capillary in origin. If bleeding continues there is probably some gum laceration or an exposed vessel in the socket. Anaesthetise the gum on either side by injecting 2 per cent lignocaine and put in a horizontal suture of nylon or silk to draw the gum margins together. If bleeding is from the socket pack it with an absorbable hydrophilic dressing (Orahesive, Squibb) or adrenaline gauze.

If the patient is a known 'bleeder' avoid suturing and seek further advice.

THE FIXED WEDDING RING

You may be faced in Casualty by a woman whose wedding ring cannot be removed from her swollen finger. Sometimes the real cause is a forgotten tight rubber band which has slipped under the ring. So look for this first. It is a pity (and difficult) to cut the ring, and the following little-known simple manoeuvre is often successful. Beginning distal to the ring wind a fine string carefully round the finger until it comes up to the ring; push the end under the ring with a matchstick, then pull gently towards the fingertip. As the string unwinds the ring comes with it.

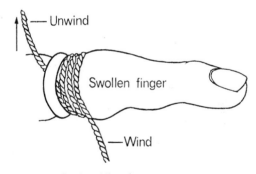

Fig. 9 How to remove a fixed wedding ring.

Rings with stones require patience and manipulation when unwinding. A little lubricant may help. A very swollen finger may be first reduced in size by injecting into it 1000 units of hyaluronidase in 1 ml of 1 g/dl lignocaine and massaging it a little. Then a length of thin rubber tubing should be wrapped round the finger from the tip up to and including the ring and left in place for five minutes. This will often reduce the swelling sufficiently to permit the ring to be drawn off or the string method to be used successfully.

NOTES ON FLUID AND ELECTROLYTES

Body fluid

The total body fluid is 60 per cent of the body weight (plasma 5 per cent; extracellular fluid 15 per cent; intracellular fluid 40 per cent).

Normal inevitable losses of fluid by an adult every 24 hours are about 1500 ml (perspiration 600 ml; expired air 400 ml; fluid to get rid of waste products in urine 500 ml). The fluid in food and produced by its oxidation roughly balance the skin and lung losses and so the urinary output usually equals the fluid drunk. Sweating, rapid breathing, youth and age increase these requirements. For safety and comfort it is best to aim at giving 3 litres of fluid every 24 hours. The adult daily requirements of sodium chloride are 80 mmol (say 4.5 g or 500 ml of isosmotic sodium chloride solution) and of potassium chloride 80 mmol (6 g).

Fluid charts

Charts of varying kinds (usually for 24 hour periods beginning at 08.00 hours) are still used in different hospitals despite the recommendations on standardisation of the Tunbridge Committee. After several days it may be difficult to get a clear picture of a patient's progress from these charts. In cases of dehydration the house physician is therefore advised to write a short statement each morning of the position up to 08.00 hours and to renew the instructions for the day.

Water depletion (results from inadequate water intake with no excessive loss of salt as in coma and high fever). Thirst. Scanty urine containing salt. No circulatory failure. Plasma sodium normal or high. Blood urea normal or slowly rising.

Salt depletion (results from excessive loss of salt with adequate water intake as in protracted vomiting, diarrhoea and Addison's disease). No thirst. Urine not scanty but free from salt (except in Addison's disease). Peripheral circulatory failure and low BP. plasma sodium low. Blood urea high (*e.g.* 15 mmol/l. Normal range 2.5–6.5 mmol/l). Patient confused, listless and later comatose.

Mixed water and salt depletion (results from excessive loss of salt and inadequate water intake as in acute vomiting). Dehydrated and thirsty. Urine scanty but salt present. Blood urea high.

How much fluid? How much salt?

These questions are best considered under two headings.

1. Prevention—how to deal with the patient in normal fluid and electrolyte balance when first seen.

2. Treatment—how to deal with the patient who is already depleted of water and electrolytes when first seen.

Prevention

Complicated electrolyte replacement is not needed at once. In each period of 24 hours a 70 kg man needs 2 to 3 litres of water. These can be given by mouth or as a rectal drip of tap water or hypotonic saline or as an i.v. drip of glucose 5 g/dl. The daily salt requirement of 4.5 g can be supplied as half a litre (one bag) of isosmotic sodium chloride solution i.v. or, if diluted, by mouth or as a rectal drip.

These considerations do not apply for the first few days after a major operation, because various factors including the endocrine response (increased secretion of adrenal cortical and pituitary antidiuretic hormones) result in a fall in the output of water and salt (and an increased loss of potassium). Water retention lasts 24 to 48 hours and salt retention three to four days. In these cases urine chloride estimations might suggest that the patient needed salt while the plasma sodium level would show that he was full of it. For the first two days after operation the fluid intake should be under 2 litres in 24 hours [say 1 litre of 5 g/dl (278 mmol/l) glucose and half a litre of isosmotic sodium chloride solution]. A urine specific gravity under 1010 is a signal to increase the saline intake. If the patient can soon take food and fluid by mouth we need not worry further but if i.v. fluid is needed for several days it may be necessary to give potassium also. A deficit should, however, be demonstrated first.

Treatment

A guide to the already dehydrated patient's need for salt (except after operation) is given by the chloride content of the urine as determined in the laboratory. If urinary chlorides are low (less than 110 mmol (4 g) per litre) or when fluid is lost by vomiting then isosmotic sodium chloride solution should be given i.v. When much saline has to be given it is well to replace one bottle in three or four by 6 mol/l sodium lactate solution to prevent acidosis. Its electrolyte content (154 mmol of Na per litre) can be regarded as the same as that of isosmotic sodium chloride solution* (160 mmol of Na per litre).

Calculation of sodium requirement

Deficit of Na = (normal level minus patient's level) × volume of body fluid

$$= (142 - \text{patient's Na level in mmol} \times 60 \text{ per cent of body weight}$$

For a 70 kg man with a plasma sodium of 118 mmol per litre;

---

*This term is used in preference to 'normal saline' (often referred to as 0.9 per cent saline) and 'physiological saline' since a chemically normal solution contains the molecular weight of a substance in grams (*e.g.* 58.5 NaCl) per litre and a truly physiological solution would contain a mixture of electrolytes.

Deficit of Na $= (142 - 118) \times \dfrac{60}{100} \times 70$

$\qquad\qquad = 24 \times 42 = 1000$ mmol Na (approx.)

One litre of isosmotic sodium chloride solution $= 160$ mmol Na (approx.). The required replacement

$= \dfrac{\text{deficit}}{160}$ litres of isosmotic sodium chloride solution

$=$ about 6½ litres

A simple formula is:

$$= \dfrac{\text{Litres of isosmotic sodium chloride solution needed}}{3}$$
$$\dfrac{142 - \text{the patient's serum sodium level in mmol}}{3}$$

A rough idea of the amount of sodium needed can be obtained by the calculation on *p* 253.

Such a calculation is only a rough guide for it is fallacious to suppose that, knowing the body weight and the plasma electrolyte levels it is possible to calculate exactly how much salt is needed to bring the plasma level back to normal. Calculations cannot allow for the state of the intracellular fluid or the efficiency of the kidneys and they ignore the adjustments which are continually taking place.

We should judge the patient's state by considering all the evidence: the history of fluid loss by vomiting, diarrhoea or through a gastric suction tube or fistula; the presence or absence of thirst; the clinical signs of dehydration (slack skin, dry tongue, soft eyeballs and collapsed veins); the urinary volume, specific gravity and chloride content and the serum sodium and potassium levels.

It must be remembered too that in addition to replacement of deficits the patient must receive also his basic needs of 1.5 litres of fluid (best given as 5 g/dl glucose) and half a litre of isosmotic sodium chloride solution ($=4.5$ g NaCl).

In general it can be stated that a patient with thirst and oliguria is short of about 4 litres of fluid and if his BP is below 90 and chlorides are absent from his urine he needs 0.75 g NaCl per kg body weight (*i.e.* about 4.5 litres of isosmotic sodium chloride solution for a 60 kg man).

Potassium depletion

In sodium depletion the extracellular fluid is hypotonic and as cell membranes are relatively impermeable to electrolytes the body cannot easily correct this completely. Some potassium does pass into the plasma, however, but the kidneys cannot conserve it. The plasma

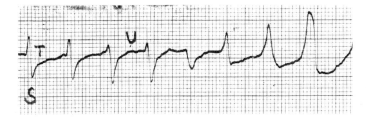

Fig. 10   Potassium deficit. (Serum level 1.5 mmol/litre.)
Low voltage, flattening of T waves. ST segment depression. Prominent U wave.
Last four complexes show probable left bundle branch block pattern due to
defective conduction. (Apparent widening of T wave sometimes seen is due to
merging of a low T wave with a U wave.)

becomes depleted and symptoms result. This possibility is increased if
potassium-free fluid is infused for several days. Suggestive symptoms
are muscular weakness, abdominal distension and mental confusion.
The e.c.g. is characteristic (Fig. 10). Unfortunately serum potassium
levels are not very reliable as an index of potassium depletion.

Treatment
Moderate potassium depletion is best corrected by giving potassium
by mouth preferably as Katorin syrup (Boots) [potassium gluconate 40
mmol (9.38 g) per 30 ml] or Slow-K tablets (Ciba) [each contains 8
mmol (600 mg) potassium chloride in a slow release base ensuring
complete absorption]. Fresh orange juice is a more natural and well-
tolerated means of giving potassium. One hundred millilitres contains
50 mmol of potassium.

When a patient can take food and fluid by mouth we need not worry
about his potassium intake but if i.v. fluid is needed for several days it
is generally necessary to give potassium. It is best not to give
potassium until water and sodium deficits are corrected and the
urinary output is good.

When i.v. replacement is needed the solution used should not
exceed 40 mmol per litre. This is achieved by adding 20 ml of
Potassium Chloride Injection BP to each litre of infused fluid. (*Note*.
This solution is too strong to give undiluted but Potassium Chloride
and Dextrose Injection BPC contains 40 mmol of K ions per litre and
can be given undiluted): any extra fluid needed should be given as 5
g/dl glucose.

Another plan is to inject potassium chloride into the bottle. Not
more than 1.5 g of potassium chloride should be put into half a litre
since this strength (40 mmol per litre) is the maximum safe strength
for i.v. administration. The rate of administration should not exceed

12 mmol per hour. A pharmacy additive service is preferable and should be used wherever possible. Commercial preparations containing 20 and 40 mmol/l are now widely employed.

Potassium intoxication

This results from excessive i.v. medication particularly if there is also renal failure. It causes weakness, flaccid paralysis and paraesthesiae. The e.c.g. shows characteristic changes (Fig. 11). Sudden death may occur from cardiac arrest even when the patient does not appear very ill. The lethal level is 10 mmol per litre. Treatment is to promote diuresis by i.m. frusemide (Lasix) injections and to reduce the extracellular potassium by causing increased cellular uptake. This is done by giving insulin and glucose (0.25 unit of insulin for each gram of glucose *e.g.* 10 units neutral insulin and 40 g glucose i.v.).

Dehydration in children

Infants have a water turnover five times greater than adults because their greater metabolism means more waste products have to pass through their relatively inefficient kidneys. A chloride output of 55 to 83 mmol per litre is normal for a child.

Type of fluid

Never use full strength isosmotic sodium chloride solution for an infant. Give it at half strength in glucose 4 g/dl or use half strength Hartmann's solution (Compound Sodium Lactate Injection BP 1958). The proprietary preparation Dioralyte (Armour) for oral use conforms to BPC recommendations. The contents of one sachet are added to 200 ml of water.

How much fluid?

The daily fluid requirements of *normal* children are:

During the first year—155 ml per kg of 'expected' body weight.

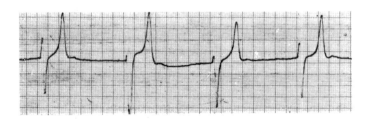

Fig. 11 Hyperkalaemia. Lead II. Increase of QRS interval. Tall peaked T waves. No evidence of atrial activity. Serum level 9.2 mmol/l.

At 3 years—1000 to 1500 ml.

At 8 years—1500 to 1900 ml.

At 12 years—2000 ml.

A dehydrated child needs *extra* fluid the amount being,

$$\frac{\text{Difference between actual and expected weight}}{\text{Expected weight}} \times \text{expected requirements}$$

Example. Expected weight 8 kg. Actùal weight 6 kg. Difference = 2.

Expected requirements 155×8=1240 ml.

Extra fluid needed is 2/8 of 1240=310 ml.

Route. By mouth if possible. Otherwise i.v. or subcutaneously with hyaluronidase 1500 units injected into the tubing.

Rate of drip. The average drip bulb *kept* at one drop per second should deliver 3 ml per minute or 180 ml per hour since the size of the average drop is 1/20 ml. As the head of pressure falls and the drip slows the actual amount delivered will be less. One drop every three seconds (60 ml per hour) is fast enough to start with. The rate should be cut down after an hour or so. Drops vary in size. The faster the drip rate the larger the drop and so doubling the drip rate more than doubles the rate at which the patient receives a drug by i.v. drip. The Tekmar volumetric drip device measures out the volume given irrespective of the drop size and composition of the fluid.

ADDISONIAN CRISIS

This may present in a previously undiagnosed patient or may follow infection or operation in a known case. The picture is that of weakness, vomiting, hypotension and pigmentation. Plasma sodium is low and the blood urea high. Estimation of plasma cortisol is essential if differentiation has to be made from salt-losing nephritis. Give 2 to 3 litres of glucose saline i.v. in 24 hours. Add to it hydrocortisone giving 100 mg every 8 hours. Give fludrocortisone 2 mg by mouth but if vomiting prevents this inject deoxycortone acetate (DOCA) 10 mg i.m. Oral management is generally possible after 24 hours. The precipitating cause, *e.g.* infection, must be treated.

ACUTE RENAL FAILURE

When oliguria or anuria presents acutely you must first try to decide whether the cause is prerenal, postrenal or renal, *i.e.* due to intrinsic renal disease. This is not as easy as one might expect but a urine urea of over 340 mmol/l suggests that the kidneys are normal.

Prerenal oliguria may be due to dehydration or failure of perfusion of the kidneys, the commonest reason being inadequate replacement of fluid following operation. So check the fluid chart and ensure that all losses are replaced. Other causes are haemorrhage and Gram-negative septicaemia. Frusemide and a 15 g mannitol infusion may be effective and if these fail acute tubular necrosis may result.

Having excluded pre- and postrenal causes the problem is to tide the patient over until renal function returns. The diagnosis of acute renal failure is indicated by resistance to frusemide, a urine/plasma osmolality ratio of less than 1.05, and a urine/plasma urea ratio less than 10. The urinary output will be low (less than 500 ml/day).

Table 6 Some 'second grade' emergencies

Clinical finding	Possible sequel of inaction	Course of action
Temporal arteritis	Retinal involvement with blindness	Steroids
Oliguria	Fits	Stop water intake
Depression	Suicide	Antidepressants ?ECT
?Pulmonary TB	Infection of others	Sputum, chest X-ray
Rose spots	Confused evidence of typhoid	Ring with Biro to identify crops
Geographic history suggesting malaria (falciparum)	Coma	Blood film and expert Chloroquine
Deep vein thrombosis	Pulmonary embolism	Anticoagulants
Purpura	Massive haemorrhage ? intracranial	Withdraw drugs, steroids
Tremor and mood changes in cirrhosis	Hepatic coma	Protein-free diet, neomycin
Salicylate overdose but patient looks well	Death	Gastric lavage
? Drug effects (*e.g.* phenothiazine rigidity)	Loss of evidence because drug eliminated	Blood and urine samples
Renal colic after cytotoxic antitumour treatment	Obstructive anuria	Increase fluid Bicarbonate Allopurinol
Oral thrush	Monilial colitis	Oral nystatin
Unusual injury in a child	Further battery	Admission Social investigation

Transfer to a haemodialysis unit should be made. While this is being arranged peritoneal dialysis (p 90) may be started and the patient put on a regime to conserve renal function. Give 500 ml of a 50 g per dl solution of glucose by central venous pressure line (p 00) and 30 units of insulin every 24 hours. A dry diet can contain up to 35 g protein. Fluid entering the mouth must be limited to 300 ml per day (plus mouth washes). As dialysed patients are liable to thrush it is well to give nystatin 100 000 units per day by mouth. Serum potassium levels must be carefully watched and prompt treatment given for any hyperkalaemia (p 256).

'SECOND GRADE' EMERGENCIES

While much of your work is not urgent you will soon realise that many conditions demand immediate attention if disaster is to be avoided. These 'second grade' emergencies are all situations which may soon become urgent unless their significance is recognised. Some examples are listed in Table 6 to help you think about this aspect of your work. It should not be forgotten that the prescription of certain drugs may place your patient in the second grade emergency category since if they should be omitted abruptly urgent symptoms of a first grade emergency could arise. Clonidine (Catapres), if withdrawn suddenly, may result in rebound hypertension with encephalopathy. Propranolol withdrawal can, over the following 10 to 14 days cause life-threatening situations such as ventricular arrhythmias and myocardial infarction.

COMA

When coma is the presenting symptom you will generally see the patient in the receiving room. Use a commonsense approach. The police or relatives or a Medic-Alert bracelet may provide the diagnosis at once. Answers to the following three questions will usually point to the cause.

1. Is there a previous history of disease which might cause coma? For example: diabetes (test urine for ketone bodies); insulin coma (if suspected give glucose 10 g i.v. *see* p 265); nephritis (test urine for albumin); falciparum malaria (make thick and thin blood films).

2. Does the immediate past history point to the cause? For example: injury (do not too readily assume that is the whole cause); poisoning (including alcohol); epilepsy (fits may be symptomatic of other disease—cerebral tumour or abscess and meningitis).

3. Are there any physical signs of disease in the central nervous system? For example: of cerebral vascular accidents and meningitis.

Normally head movements cause conjugate movements of the eyes to the opposite side. Failure to show these 'doll's head eye movements' argues in favour of organic brain disease. Failure of syringing an ear with iced water to cause deviation of the eyes to the irrigated side has similar significance.

Always make a full examination and record the findings. These must include the urine, pupils, fundi, heart rate, blood pressure and temperature. If hypoglycaemia is a possibility an exception to the advice (*p* 265) to give glucose i.v. is the rare case of Wernicke's encephalopathy which glucose would worsen. (Thiamine would be indicated).

Beware of saying a patient is only drunk and handing him over to the police when he might have a head injury also (*see p* 58).

Management of the comatose patient
Three aspects of prolonged coma require careful management.

1. *Adequate oxygenation.* Preserve the airway and use artificial respiration if need be, *i.e.* if the rate and depth of breathing is no more than enough to clear the dead space so that cyanosis results.

2. *Position.* The correct position lessens the risk of aspiration pneumonia and should be maintained until the patient can cough and swallow properly. Place the patient on his side and with the foot of the bed raised 15 to 25 cm. Put pillows behind his back and between his knees but not under his head. Adhesive felt should protect the shoulder.

3. *Fluid balance.* An adult should receive 2500 ml of fluid (5 g/dl glucose) and 4.5 g sodium chloride each day by intragastric or i.v. drip. A calorie intake of 1500 should be aimed at.

Watch your word
Don't talk too freely at the bedside lest you cause distress. Your 'comatose' patient may be more alert than you think. In the rare 'locked-in syndrome' a pontine lesion renders your patient quadriplegic though alert and sentient. Some voluntary eyelid opening movements remain. So beware of saying unwise things in the belief that the patient cannot hear them. Remember too that hearing is the last conscious function to disappear under anaesthesia and may reappear early during recovery from circulatory arrest.

NOTES ON DIABETES

Diagnosis
This is proved by a random blood sugar level two hours after a meal of

10 mmol/l or more. If necessary a glucose tolerance test should be done (*p* 213).

Diet

Only the carbohydrate content of a diet is fixed nowadays. The protein and fat are free except when, in obese diabetics, the total calorie intake must be fixed also. The intelligent diabetic has considerable choice from his list of portions of foods containing 10 g carbohydrate and if need be a list of calorie values (*p* 60). He can buy a Diabetic Association booklet showing the composition of proprietary foods. The dietitian or nurse will teach the patient about his diet, how to test urine and how to use his insulin (BS 1619) syringe. A rough rule is that the carbohydrate in grams × 10 shows the calorie intake when the patient chooses usual portions of fat and protein.

Drinks

Spirits, dry sherry and red wine (but not port) may be taken since they contain little or no carbohydrate. Half an ounce (15 g) of bread should be omitted for every half pint (300 ml) of beer or cider taken and for each small bottle of tonic water or lemon drink. For more detailed information about the carbohydrate content of alcoholic drinks see leaflet DH122 of the British Diabetic Association.

Tablets

Some obese diabetics are controlled by a daily diet of 100 g carbohydrate and 1000 calories. If this is insufficient add a sulphonylurea drug chlorpropamide (Diabinese) 100 mg before breakfast.

In the non-obese diabetic if carbohydrate restriction is not enough give chlorpropamide (Diabinese) 250 mg before breakfast adding metformin (Glucophage) 850 mg twice daily if necessary. Failure of diet and tablets calls for insulin.

Insulin

You should make yourself familiar with the various insulins and the colour code for identification. Monocomponent insulins (highly purified beef and pork preparations) are replacing older types. Examples include Actrapid (neutral insulin) (duration of action about 7 hours) and Monotard MC (Insulin Zinc Suspension BP) which lasts about 16 hours. On change over to a monocomponent insulin the dose should be reduced by 15 per cent.

A patient on insulin should distribute his carbohydrate so that in addition to the usual four meals he also takes 10 or 20 g carbohydrate for 'elevenses' and for a night cap. You will learn how to prescribe insulin from practical experience. Do not be discouraged if at first the patients know more about it than you do. Severe and complicated diabetes and diabetes in pregnancy call for two daily injections of insulin. Make any increment or reduction of insulin at least one-fifth of the previous dose. The effect of smaller changes is inappreciable. 'Brittle' diabetics whose blood sugar swings widely need NPH insulin as well as neutral insulin the dose of each being adjusted by urine tests.

If changing from two or more daily injections of neutral insulin or one dose of PZI plus soluble a good rule is to give three-quarters of the previous total daily dose of neutral insulin as Monotard and add to it half the previous morning dose of neutral insulin. A daily dose of 12 units or less can be replaced entirely by Monotard.

At the follow-up clinic. All urine tests should be made on short term specimens, *i.e.* on urine passed half an hour after emptying the bladder. Tell the patient to bring three specimens to the clinic:

1. passed half an hour before supper (having emptied the bladder of urine half an hour earlier and discarded it);
2. passed just before breakfast (having discarded the specimen passed on rising);
3. urine passed just before the midday meal (having emptied the bladder an hour earlier).

He should label each specimen with his name and the time when it was passed.

Capillary blood glucose measurement at home (using simplified reflectometers and Dextrostix) in suitable cases is now advocated so as to achieve better control.

Diabetic ketoacidosis (pre-coma)

This is shown by ketonuria plus symptoms (anorexia, overbreathing and drowsiness).

Give Actrapid (neutral insulin) as a continuous infusion. Twenty-four units are diluted to 20 ml with isosmotic sodium chloride solution in a 20 ml syringe fitted to a Handley infusion pump. The infusion rate will be about 2 units of Actrapid per hour. Low dose i.m. insulin can be used in very restless patients. In addition give liquid carbohydrate 20 g every 2 hours (or i.v. if vomiting) until the urine is ketone-free. This usually takes 24 hours.

(Carbohydrate 10 g is contained in two lumps of sugar, 120 ml orange juice, 210 ml milk and two teaspoonsful of Benger's food, Horlicks milk or Ovaltine.)

Look carefully for any infection which might have caused ketosis.

Diabetic coma (with ketoacidosis)

This is now less common than it was. The problem of ketosis is complicated by dehydration and, because of unconsciousness, by inability to drink. Average losses have been estimated as: water 6 litres; sodium 500 mmol; potassium 350 mmol; phosphate 75 mmol; and magnesium 20 mmol.

Aspirate the stomach (*see p* 78) and check that the urine output is adequate. Give 6 units of neutral insulin hourly by continuous infusion. The blood sugar will fall by about 5 mmol per litre per hour. Occasionally more insulin is needed. Reduce to 2 units per hour when the blood sugar is between 10 and 15 mmol/l. Maintain the blood sugar concentration around 5 to 10 mmol/l by adjusting the amount of insulin infused, until the patient is able to eat. Then give the usual morning or evening dose of insulin followed 30 minutes later by 40 g carbohydrate as a small meal. If this is retained discontinue insulin and dextrose infusion (*vide infra*). Sliding scale 4-hourly subcutaneous neutral insulin is used when the daily insulin requirement has not been previously established.

One litre of isosmotic sodium chloride solution is given during the first hour followed by up to 2.5 litres over the next 5 hours. When the blood glucose level reaches 15 mmol/l change to 5 g/dl dextrose (6 g per hour). Infuse potassium when the plasma level is below 6 mmol/l (initially 13 mmol/hour reducing to 5 mmol/hour). Monitor plasma potassium levels. Commence oral potassium supplements after the 40 g carbohydrate meal and continue for one week.

After recovery persuade the patient to join the British Diabetic Association if he is not already a member.

Never forget that a diabetic may become unconscious from causes unconnected with his diabetes (*see* Table 7).

Diabetic coma (without ketoacidosis). Hyperosmolar coma

This occurs in elderly patients not previously known to be diabetic but with a short history of thirst and polyuria. The high blood sugar (55 mmol or more per litre) causes an osmotic diuresis. Treatment is to give half strength isosmotic sodium chloride solution i.v. changing to 2.5 g/dl glucose as the blood sugar falls. Insulin should be given cautiously and in smaller doses than the high blood sugar would suggest for there is a real danger of hypoglycaemia with big doses. As arterial thrombosis is a frequent complication anticoagulant therapy should be started. Probably there are many syndromes in which

Table 7 Cause of coma in a diabetic

Cause of coma	Colour	Breathing	Eyes	Tongue	Glycosuria	Ketosis	Babinski's sign
Ketosis	Flushed	Air hunger. Acetone in breath	Soft	Dry	++++	++++	→
Hypoglycaemia	Pale (Sweating)	Normal	Normal	Moist	Probably nil	Nil	↑
Stroke	Flushed or pale	Stertorous or Cheyne-Stokes	Pupillary changes	Normal	May be +	Nil	↑
Drugs	Varies	Slow and shallow	May be small pupils	Normal	Nil	Nil	May be ↑
hyper-osmolarity	Varies	No change	Soft	Dry	++++	Slight or absent	→

hyperosmolarity plays a part. A similar picture can complicate peritoneal dialysis when the fluid used contains glucose.

Hypoglycaemia

All diabetics on insulin should be given an overdose in order to learn what they feel like when hypoglycaemic. They should all carry six lumps of sugar (5 g carbohydrate in each) to take if an attack threatens. The rapid onset of coma in a diabetic suggests hypoglycaemia. You will not find the differentiation from diabetic coma difficult except in the partially treated patient when reliance must be placed on blood sugar estimations. If in doubt take blood for blood glucose or use Dextrostix at the bedside but do not wait for the result. Glucose i.v. can do no harm and if there is any doubt about diagnosis give it first.

A 20 ml syringeful of glucose 50 g/dl will promptly bring round all but the most severe case of hypoglycaemic coma.

A very effective alternative is glucagon 0.2 ml per kg i.m. or i.v. If the hypoglycaemic patient is having a long-acting insulin, *e.g.* Monotard or chlorpropamide, do not send him home at once on recovery as he may relapse. (Hypoglycaemia may cause hemiparesis, reversible with glucose, in elderly patients).

HYPOTHERMIA

A low body temperature may not be registered if the thermometer is used incorrectly. A notch at the base of the column prevents the mercury falling and so it is essential first to shake the mercury down below the scale. If the mercury does not reach this the temperature is below 35°C and a special low-reading rectal thermometer must be used. In hypothermia the abdomen and axillae, normally always warm, are cold to the touch.

The elderly hypothermic patient (temperature below 32.2°C) may have reached this state because a stroke, fracture or infection has made him immobile. Sometimes drugs (phenothiazines and barbiturates) are a factor. The picture may resemble myxoedema. Active rewarming is harmful (except in the young). Put the patient in a warm room under a single blanket. Start a slow glucose infusion. A broad-spectrum antibiotic should be started. Hypoxia and acidosis call for corrective measures. Hydrocortisone 100 mg 8 hourly i.v. is helpful but only when there is definite myxoedema, which hypothermia may resemble, should specific treatment for it be given. Then use tri-iodothyronine 5μg every hour by slow i.v. drip and start thyroxine 0.1 mg daily.

POISONING

Advice may be obtained at any time from the official Poisons Information Centres:

London   01-407 7600
Edinburgh   031-229 2477
Cardiff   (0222) 49223
Belfast   (0232) 40503
Dublin   45588.

There are several unofficial poisons centres which will give advice:

Consett, Co Durham, Shotley Bridge Hospital; (020 72) 3456 Ext 57
Leeds   (0532) 32799
Brandon, Suffolk, 48th Tactical Hospital, RAF Lakenheath; (0638 81) 2666
Romford   (70) 46099
Manchester   061-740 2254

Suspect poisoning or overdosage in any obscurely comatose patient. Identify any tablets found (*see p* 231).

The general principles of treatment are to remove or neutralise the poison and to keep the patient alive by dealing with whatever state is most threatening life. These measures are more important than the use of antidotes except in those cases where there is a very specific one and the poison is known, *e.g.* desferrioxamine for iron poisoning.

The stomach should be washed out:

1. If the patient is seen within four hours of swallowing tablets (unless only a few were taken).

2. If the patient is unconscious and the time of taking the tablets is unknown.

3. In all cases of salicylate poisoning.

Gastric lavage (*p* 78) is generally contraindicated if corrosive poison has been swallowed though its risk has to be weighed against that of absorption of the poison. When kerosene or petrol is swallowed by a child lavage is risky. If the stomach must be emptied it is better to use ipecac. Keep any vomit and the first washings for analysis. If you have no tube and gastric emptying is imperative you may give a conscious adult patient apomorphine 6 mg i.v. and sit him up. It should never be given to a comatose patient for his vomiting centre is too depressed to respond and the drug may then depress other centres. [Antidote: naloxone (Narcan) 1 ml ampoule (0.4 mg).] (For use of ipecac in a child, *see p* 79.)

Haemo- or peritoneal dialysis may be arranged to remove dialysable substances if their blood levels warrant this.

Aspirin poisoning

Since salicylate is held in the stomach for long periods gastric emptying by syringe or Señorans's evacuator followed by gastric lavage should always be performed. Renal excretion of salicylate is enhanced in an alkaline urine but oral alkaline fluids are insufficient. Forced alkaline diuresis should be started if the plasma level is 3.6 mmol/l or more (2.2 mmol/l in children) or without this estimation if the clinical state looks serious. The risk of causing serious hypokalaemia is avoided by the 'cocktail' diuresis described by Lawson *et al.* (*Quarterly Journal of Medicine,* 1969, **149,** 31) which renders biochemical control unnecessary. Give the following solution i.v. at the rate of 2 litres per hour for three hours:

> Saline (154 mmol/l) 0.5 litre
> Laevulose (278 mmol/l) 1.0 litre
> Sodium bicarbonate (150 mmol/l) 0.5 litre
> Potassium chloride 40 mmol

Infusion should go on until the plasma salicylate level is below 2.2 mmol per litre. Renal function must be adequate.

Paracetamol (Panadol) poisoning
The chief risk caused by overdosage by this common analgesic is of severe delayed liver damage but this is unlikely if the plasma level is below 1.3 mmol/l four hours after ingestion. When hepatic toxicity is probable give Parvolex (Duncan Flockhart) (200 mg N-cysteine per ml). The initial dose is 150 mg/kg. It is ineffective after 15 hours (*see* literature). Keep the urine. See Acute Liver Injury (*p* 245).

Distalgesic poisoning
As this proprietary tablet contains dextropropoxyphene (Doloxene) as well as paracetamol even a small overdose can rapidly cause coma and apnoea especially˙ if taken with alcohol. Naloxone (Narcan) and artificial respiration will be needed as well as treatment as for paracetamol poisoning.

Paraquat poisoning (Weedol etc.)
Empty the stomach. Give repeated doses of a suspension of Fuller's earth. Start forced diuresis with frusemide 40 mg i.v. Ask a Poisons Information Centre (*p* 266) re 19 special Paraquat Centres with a view to charcoal haemo-perfusion. Keep the urine.

Barbiturate poisoning

Wash out the stomach if seen within four hours or if unconscious and the time of taking tablets is not known. Mild cases need nursing and supportive measures only. Maintain respiration—artificially if need be. Set up a 5 g/dl dextrose drip (2 litres in 24 hours). Combat shock by head-down tilt. Make the urine alkaline by giving 230 mg per kg BW sodium bicarbonate as Injection of Sodium Bicarbonate BP 5 g/dl (595 mmol/l). Consider haemoperfusion in severe cases.

Antidotes

For morphine poisoning use naloxone (Narcan) 0.4 to 1.2 mg i.v. in divided doses. It also antagonises pethidine and methadone (Physeptone) but not barbiturates. Its action is brief (half life 20 min).

For cyanide poisoning use amyl nitrite by inhalation and cobalt EDTA (Kelocyanor) 20 ml (300 mg) i.v.

For mercury poisoning use BAL (Dimercaprol) 300 mg i.m. and then 150 mg four hourly.

Should you tell the police? No; attempted suicide is no longer an indictable offence so there is now no legal obligation to report it to the police. Steps to avoid a further attempt—such as moving the patient away from an upstairs window—would be wise.

Food poisoning

Bacterial food poisons. Symptoms within two to four hours after eating. Usually cream cake or trifle containing staphylococcal toxin.

Bacterial food infections. Symptoms more than 12 hours after eating. Often caused by manipulated meats (salmonella organisms).

Note the foods eaten; take charge of any remains; save vomit and faeces and notify the community physician. Do not ask for agglutination tests until the stools have been cultured or in any case during the first week.

Treatment

Vomiting may be induced by putting two fingers down the throat after a drink of bicarbonate but it is unwise to wash out the stomach. Secure adequate hydration by fruit and effervescent drinks. An i.v. drip may be necessary. Diphenoxylate with atropine (Lomotil) 2.5 mg tablets (10 to 15 mg in 24 hours) often helps as does Kaolin and Morphine Mixture BNF 15 ml four-hourly. Antibiotics and especially cotrimoxazole (Bactrim, Septrin) should be avoided as they can produce faecal carriers. Even if there is toxaemia and probable bloodstream invasion chloramphenicol should not be given unless the condition is typhoid.

Don't be persuaded to certify 'Food poisoning' until this is proved. A certificate may be wanted simply to blackmail a restaurant.

Poisonous plants

You may be faced in Casualty by an anxious parent who says her child has eaten some berries. Of the 200 British plants which have poisonous constituents only a few cause serious illness. If you can see and identify the berries and can consult HM Stationery Office publication *British Poisonous Plants* you may be able to reassure the parents. All that can be said here is that the following berries are harmless: cotoneaster, pyracantha, hawthorn, lily of the valley, nasturtium and sweet pea. Yew seeds and other parts of the tree are very dangerous. Treatment is on general lines by gastric emptying, artificial respiration and the control of convulsions. (Have the tree cut down.) For deadly nightshade poisoning empty the stomach and give the antidote neostigmine (Prostigmin) 0.5 to 1.0 mg i.m.

The rare emergency of 'mushroom' poisoning is treated on general lines unless the cause is thought to be the 'Death Cap' (*Amanita phalloides*). Confirm this by (a) examining uneaten fungi (the death cap has white gills), (b) noting the 12-hour interval before symptoms begin, (c) sending vomit and faeces for spores. If death cap poisoning is proven or probable empty the stomach (*p* 78) and offer this treatment to all those who have shared the meal irrespective of whether they have symptoms or not. Arrange early charcoal haemoperfusion.

THE RED EYE

The patient with a red eye presents the house physician with a worrying problem. If in serious doubt he should seek expert advice. Table 8 will help him to decide. It is good practice to use a drop of 1 g/dl amethocaine hydrochloride to facilitate examination of a painful eye.

SPONTANEOUS PNEUMOTHORAX

Confirm your clinical suspicions by a chest X-ray film taken in expiration. A small pneumothorax calls for no special measures. A completely collapsed lung demands active treatment to hasten its otherwise slow re-expansion. Watch carefully in the first few hours for signs of internal haemorrhage and evidence of fluid as well as air. Sometimes a slow drip of blood from the parietal end of a torn adhesion fills the pleural space with blood. (Should this happen start a

Table 8 The red eye

Symptom or sign	Conjunctivitis	Keratitis	Iritis	Glaucoma
Discharge	+	Watering only	Watering only	Watering only
Pain	Discomfort only	+	++	+++ and vomiting
Vision	Normal	Depends on how much opacity covers the pupil	Reduced	Greatly reduced
Congestion	Conjunctival	Ciliary	Ciliary	Ciliary
Corneal transparency	Normal	Localised opacity	General haze	General clouding
Anterior chamber	Normal	Normal	Normal	Shallow
Iris and pupil	Normal reactions	Small and reacts to light	Small and bound down. Reflexes may be absent	No reaction to light
Tension	Normal	Normal	Perhaps a little increased	Greatly increased
The other eye	Often affected also	Old scars of previous ulcers	May be old iritis with bound down pupil	May be cupped disc

transfusion and send for a surgeon. Open thoracotomy is the best way of dealing with the problem.) Plastic tubes with introducers are now available. Insert one in the 3rd or 4th intercostal space in the midaxillary line and connect it to a glass tube which dips into 500 ml of water in a large bottle. The depth below the surface is adjusted so that bubbles of air can be expelled on deep expiration. This device ensures that air cannot be drawn into the chest via the tube. When the tube has to be adjusted it should be clamped near to the chest first. Your chief may like to apply continuous suction in these cases and then you should attach a manometer to a side arm. It is best to use a small electric pump adjusted so that its maximum suction capacity does not exceed the upper limit of the suction you want. Another simple method is to connect a large bottle of water to the chest catheter and let water drip slowly from a bottom outlet. The tube's position and the subsequent resorption of gas should be confirmed radiologically. Failure of reduction in size of the pneumothorax suggests a broncho-pleural fistula. A sample of gas drawn from it into a special tube by displacement of mercury will show a high oxygen content (=alveolar air). There is little oxygen left in a closed pneumothorax after a few hours.

Tension pneumothorax. When a valvular mechanism allows air entering the pleural space to be trapped there tension builds up. Mediastinal displacement and impaired venous return quickly result. Deal with this emergency by prompt insertion of a needle or thoracic catheter. A punctured rubber glove finger tied over the needle or preferably a proper flutter valve will ensure that air leaks but does not re-enter the pleural space.

ARTIFICIAL RESPIRATION

If breathing has stopped for ten minutes death is almost certain and it may occur after a two minute stoppage. So when breathing fails artificial respiration must be started *on the spot* at once. *There is literally not one second to lose.* Don't stop to remove dentures, to loosen clothing or drain the lungs. All these can be attended to later.

The best method is direct insufflation of the patient's lungs with your expired air, an ancient method of mouth-to-mouth resuscitation mentioned in the Bible (II Kings IV. 34) and therefore called 'Elisha breathing' and popularly known as the 'Kiss of Life'.

Technique
Some prefer mouth-to-*nose* technique since it can be used with the patient on his side and carries less risk of inflating the stomach and

subsequent trouble from vomiting. If the mouth-to-mouth method is used the patient must be on his back. If external cardiac massage has to be done at the same time, it is an advantage to have the patient off the ground on a hard surface. This position also facilitates laryngeal intubation should it become necessary. It is very important to align the pharynx and larynx correctly (Fig. 12). Using both hands lift the head (A) and tilt it back (B). You may put your thumb in the victim's mouth to grasp the jaw if need be. Put your lips over the patient's mouth or nose (or mouth and nose in a child) so as to make a good seal. With the thumb and forefinger of one hand close the patient's nostrils or lips gently (a nose clip may be used). Take a deep breath and exhale into the patient (with a few puffs in the newborn). You should see and feel the chest rise. Then remove your lips and let the chest deflate.

Those who have used this method say that in the thrill of the emergency they do not find it repulsive but some are happier if they avoid contact with the patient and breathe into the hole of an oronasal mask or a simple device, the Resusciade, a nylon mouthpiece with a valve set in a small sheet of plastic. A Brook airway (Fig. 13) is probably the best appliance to use. During expiration a valve closes the blow tube and allows air to escape by a side vent. The tube prevents the tongue from falling back. Air blown into the stomach may cause an

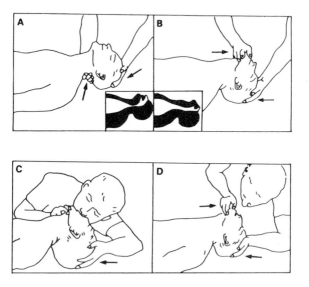

Fig. 12 Artificial respiration. Head-tilt oral method. A, neck is lifted; B, head is fully tilted back; C, lungs are inflated via nose or mouth; and D, victim exhales by himself, if necessary through his mouth. (By courtesy of the Editor of the *Journal of the American Medical Association*.)

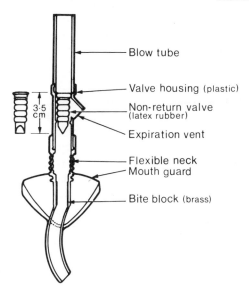

Blow tube

Valve housing (plastic)

Non-return valve
(latex rubber)

3·5
cm

Expiration vent

Flexible neck
Mouth guard

Bite block (brass)

Fig. 13 The Brook airway.

explosive vomit which will threaten the air passages. Be ready to clear the pharynx by suction. A similar but simpler (valveless) resuscitation tube is the SALAD* airway. Its long end is inserted in adults and its short end in children. Repeat the cycle 12 times a minute turning your head away as you breathe in so as not to fill your lungs with the patient's expired air. Continue inflation and deflation of the lungs until spontaneous breathing is maintained.

Overvigorous use of artificial respiration may wash out CO_2 from the blood and so remove the normal stimulus to breathing. This may account for those cases in which recovery of breathing has been delayed for many hours although the pulse has returned and the colour is good. In none of the methods should the frequency be more than 12 per minute. Another risk is gastric inflation followed by vomiting and inhalation of stomach contents. It can be avoided by seeing that inflation is unhurried and not too forceful. Excessive pressure sufficient to inflate the stomach is less likely in mouth-to-nose than in mouth-to-mouth inflation.

The advantages of this method are that it is universally applicable and that it leaves both hands free to control the jaw and maintain an airway. A possible disadvantage is that the 4 to 5 per cent of CO_2 in the operator's expired air may be deleterious to the hypoxic and hypercap-

*Save A Life A Day Campaign, 9 Whitecliff Road, Parkstone, Poole, Dorset BH14 8DU Price 72p plus postage.

nic patient. This would only be important if artificial respiration was prolonged and could be avoided by interposing a CO_2 absorber between the operator and the victim.

How long to go on
Continue mouth-to-mouth artificial respiration until natural breathing is permanently restored (stop every 10 minutes to see) or death is diagnosed by absence of heart beats (or no e.c.g. signs) for 5 minutes. When the heart beats continue but breathing is maintained by machine the decision to switch off, though not urgent, should be achieved soon for it is bad for morale to continue hopelessly and unfair to the relatives to let them hope in vain for survival (*see* Brain Death, *p* 11). To give the patient a chance to return to consciousness all drugs should be stopped for two to seven days. In certain cases (hypothermia, barbiturate poisoning, drowning and electrocution) IPPV should go on longer than in other cases. An e.e.g. may help one to decide but a decision to switch off should not be made simply because the record is flat.

CIRCULATORY ARREST

Try to see one of the excellent films showing the technique of cardiac compression and make yourself familiar with the 'May Day' procedure used in your hospital. You will not be called to patients whose cardiac arrest is merely a terminal event or to any patient for whom your chief may have decided that resuscitation would be inappropriate. You may find resuscitation already in progress. If it is not the steps you should take are:

1. Confirm that the pulse in the carotid artery is absent.
Note the time.
Do not delay to see if other pulses can be felt or listen wonderingly for heart sounds for this would waste the precious minutes during which the brain may be saved.
2. Summon assistance by sounding the 'May Day' alarm.
3. Give a sharp blow over the heart.
4. If ineffective give a defibrillating shock.
5. If ineffective (or while awaiting the defibrillator) keep the cerebral circulation going. Put a hard resuscitation board under the patient. Raise the legs. Insert a Brook or other airway and start cardiac compression manually (60 compressions a minute). Until help arrives you will have to stop once every 15 compressions to inflate the lungs twice by mouth. You will also have to pause occasionally to see if spontaneous beating has returned. If you are easily fatigued you could

put the victim on the flóor and use the ball of your foot instead of your hands.

6. Ask someone to give 100 ml of $NaHCO_3$ 8.4 g/dl i.v. (100mmol).

7. If e.c.g. shows simple asystole give 10 ml calcium chloride $CaCl_2$ $2H_2O$ 13.4 g/dl and 10 ml 1 in 10000 adrenaline into the L ventricle. Enter a long needle near the apex beat. (Bleeding is less likely than when the R atrium is entered). Failing this inject an arm vein and flush it through. For recurring bouts of ventricular fibrillation give 1 or 2 mg of lignocaine by drip per minute.

8. Check the blood gases and pH.

9. Start measures to combat cerebral oedema. Give dexamethasone 4 mg i.v. Failing this use frusemide 2 ml i.v.

Note on defibrillation
An effective shock will make the trunk muscles contract. There is a risk of giving a shock to bystanders so no one should be touching the patient when the shock is given. Cardiac compression and artificial respiration must continue between shocks if several are needed. Avoidable reasons for failure are:

1. Broken wires, wrong adaptors, etc., avoidable by regular checking.
2. Incorrect placement of electrodes. One should be on the right sternal border and the other on the left side of the heart.
3. Short circuiting by excess of electrode paste.
4. Insufficient energy. For persons over 50 kg 400 joules are needed.

How long to go on
If you are the first person on the scene you will have to continue the cardiac compression already started. Ten minutes is about the limit of one's endurance for cardiac compression and an assistant or machine should be ready to take over then or earlier. But the circulation must be kept going until skilled help including a defibrillator arrives. After the slightest flicker of encouragement rhythmic compression should continue for an hour or until the heart beat is established. If there has been no suggestion of a heart beat or an effective return of circulation as shown by an improvement in colour, constriction of the pupils and a carotid pulse for an hour despite treatment the situation is hopeless. An e.c.g. may help (test it on a volunteer to make sure it is working). If the circulation is maintained but the patient remains comatose and needs artificial respiration, this should go on for four to eight hours before being abandoned. If there is a chance of organ transplantation, however, artificial respiration must to on until a decision is reached. If the question of transplant surgery does not arise the decision to switch

off the respirator should be made by the most experienced doctors present.

Cardiac pacing

Once the HP has become familiar with the apparatus and has witnessed its insertion it is within his competence to use it. The major indication is complete heart block with frequent Stokes-Adams' episodes. Pacing is often a temporary measure used until full recovery occurs following cardiac infarction. It may have to be used pending the insertion of a permanent pacemaker. Although it can be performed 'blind' via the internal jugular vein or a vein in the antecubital fossa it is best to use the subclavian vein guided by an image intensifier.

Always check that all equipment is in order and wear a lead apron. An apprehensive patient may be helped by diazepam (Valium) 5-10 mg i.v.

Proceed as described for subclavian venepuncture (*p* 86). The 5F USCI pacing electrode will pass easily through the Medicut 14 g cannula. Using the image intensifier guide the tip into the right atrium and form a loop. Rotate the electrode and advance it through the tricuspid valve until it lies on the floor of the right ventricle with its tip at the apex of the ventricle (anterior position in the lateral view). Connect the wire marked 'distal' (from the electrode tip) to 'Active' and that marked 'proximal' (1 cm back from the electrode tip) to 'Indifferent' on the temporary external pacing box. Set the pacing stimulus to 3 volts and its rate faster than the natural one. Switch the pacemaker to give 'demand' pacing. Make sure the pacing threshold is below 1 volt and that the ventricular response is not interrupted when the patient coughs or breathes deeply. The stimulus width is about 1 millisecond. Check the intravascular portion of the electrode to exclude loop formation resulting from excessive electrode rotation. This is less likely when the larger 6F electrode and 12 gauge Medicut are used. When catheter placement is satisfactory fix a loop of electrode in the infraclavicular region with a 3–0 Dexon suture.

When left in place for a few days the natural rise in threshold may exceed the pacing voltage and this may need readjustment. Prednisolone 10 mg four times a day may make the pacing threshold rise more slowly. Complete heart block following myocardial infarction may last up to three weeks before reversion to sinus rhythm occurs. Approximately 5 per cent of these cases require a permanent pacemaker.

SOME URGENT MEDICAL ACCIDENTS

Almost any of the common medical procedures you use may, on

occasion, prove hazardous. You should be aware of what might go wrong and be ready with the remedy. Here are a few reminders.

Wrong patient. Always check his name and number.

Wrong injections. Always read the label beforehand.

Broken needles. If a needle breaks and a little projects remove it with forceps. Otherwise immobilise the part and leave it alone until X-ray examination and a planned operation can be made. Tell the patient but don't admit liability. Keep the parts and report to your Medical Defence Society.

Accidental intra-arterial injection—see p 85

Accidental injection of a toxic dose. If in a limb apply a tourniquet and release momentarily at intervals. Elsewhere consider incision and apply ice. Use an antidote, *e.g.* naloxone (Narcan) for overdosage by morphine and other opiates.

ANAPHYLAXIS

See Serum administration, *p* 118

AIR EMBOLISM

If collapse follows needling of the chest air may have reached the left heart via the pulmonary veins and then the coronary arteries or brain. Withdraw the needle, lower the head and turn the patient on to his left side. The portion of the aortic orifice uppermost will then be the part which does not have a coronary orifice in it. A similar accident following injection into a peripheral vein will fill the right heart with froth (or cross to the left side by a patent foramen ovale—'paradoxical embolism'). Treat in the same way. The risk of frothy blood rising into the outflow tract of the right ventricle is lessened by lying on the left side.

BEE AND WASP STINGS

A honeybee (but not a wasp) leaves her sting in the skin. It should be scraped (not picked) out. A severe reactor shows generalised urticaria and bronchospasm; the quicker the onset the more severe the case. Put a tourniquet above the sting and loosen it every few minutes. Apply ice. You may inject adrenaline and use the other items on the anaphylaxis tray (*p* 118). A beekeeper known to react severely may carry the remedy and put a Tablet of Isoprenaline BP 10 mg (if obtainable) under the tongue. An alternative is to take three puffs of adrenaline from a Medihaler-Epi.

THE DRUG ADDICT

You should be aware of the possibility that a drug addict may present at hospital as a puzzling case of mysterious illness whose cause (drug deprivation) is not disclosed. Alternatively he may be a self-confessed addict clamouring for his drug. Most addicts take their drugs by mouth but your suspicions will be confirmed in some cases by needle puncture marks—often infected—and a puffy hand.

Some aspects of the case will help you to spot the drug. Very often more than one is being taken. Amphetamine addicts may present as violent psychiatric emergencies. An appearance as if drunk in a patient claiming sleeplessness from loss of his tablets suggests the barbiturate addict. Injections of dissolved barbiturate tablets often leave indolent ulcers. The cannabis addict rarely presents at hospital.

Management

Do not fall for a plausible story of loss of drugs and simply prescribe some more. Junkies are skilful and incorrigible liars. Put the patient where he can be observed and do not send him away. If you remain doubtful about what to do admit him until he can be seen by a consultant. Sometimes the problem is simply anxiety about further supplies of drugs. Sympathetic handling and a chance to simmer down will help. There is no withdrawal state with cannabis, amphetamine and LSD and so there is no justification for prescribing these drugs.

Heroin addicts generally congregate in London within easy reach of its treatment centres which are essentially concerned with opiates. Problems produced by other drugs should be dealt with on general lines. If you know or suspect that your patient is addicted to heroin or other opiates you must, within seven days, get in touch with the Drugs Branch of the Home Office, 50 Queen Anne's Gate, London S.W.1. (tel. *see below*) who will give you details of any known addict in the UK or Northern Ireland. When you think the symptoms are genuinely due to withdrawal of heroin you should contact the physician authorised under The Misuse of Drugs (Notification of and Supply to Addicts) Regulations 1973 and obtain his authority to give methadone 10 to 20 mg preferably as a linctus. This will relieve the symptoms for 12 hours or so. Then arrange to transfer the patient to a treatment centre of which there are 25 in Greater London and 50 elsewhere in Great Britain. The hospital administrator will have details of these and their consultants. Failing him ask the Home Office. Most are in general psychiatric clinics.

The treatment centre will want to be sure that treatment is not being already received elsewhere and so will ask the Home Office if they can identify the addict. When you ring the Drugs Branch, which is open during normal office hours, dial:

01-213 5141 for patients with surnames A to G
01-213 4274 for patients with surnames H to P
01-213 6083 for patients with surnames Q to Z
01-213 3403 for general inquiries.

Make a note of tattoos, birthmarks, scars, colour of eyes and hair, complexion and any special features. There is no reason to conceal the fact that these particulars may be used for identity check. Treatment for soft drug addiction is available at most psychiatric outpatient departments. General advice can be obtained from The Institute for the Study of Drug Dependence, Kingsbury House, 3 Blackburn Road, London NW6 1XA (tel. 01-328 5541).

WHAT TO DO WHEN THERE IS LITTLE TO BE DONE

You may be called at the instigation of the relatives to the bedside of someone dying of advanced carcinoma. While a commonplace scene to you they may never have witnessed it before. So do not show any impatience. As there will no doubt be a high tolerance of morphine there is no objection to using one of the euphoric mixtures such as:

Diamorphine hydrochloride   10 mg
Honey   4 ml
Chloroform water   to 15 ml

It is not your duty to prolong the act of dying. There is no objection to using drugs to relieve suffering even if they will indirectly hasten death, but if the patient's spiritual affairs are not in order you should hesitate to use drugs which would diminish his faculties.

Your aim should be to control all symptoms. Drugs to control pain should not be given only at timed intervals but when required and before pain recurs.

Eponymous names

Numbers after names are those of the pages on which they are mentioned.

Abrams, Leon David   90, 93, 94
Born 1923. Cardiothoracic surgeon, Birmingham, England.

Adams, Robert   276
1791–1875, Irish surgeon. President of Royal College of Surgeons of Ireland. Surgeon to Queen Victoria.

Addison, Thomas   143, 213, 257
1795–1860. Physician to Guy's Hospital, London. Discovered Addison's disease of the adrenals. The founder of endocrinology.

Ambu   110
*A*ir, *M*ask, *B*ag, *U*nit. Alternatively the first four letters of the word Ambulance.

Armstrong, Arthur Riley   143
Born 1904. Director of Laboratories, Chidoke Hospital (formerly The Mountain Sanatorium). Hamilton, Ontario, Canada.

Ayre, James Ernest   98, 138
1910–1974. Director, Papanicolaou Cancer Research Institute, Miami, Florida, USA. Originally a Canadian he worked first in Montreal.

Baker, William M.   63
1839–1896. Surgeon, St Bartholomew's Hospital, London.

Barré Jean Alexandre   212
1880–1967. Strasbourg neurologist.

Bilharz, Theodor   65
1825–1862. Born in Württemberg. Professor of Anatomy in Cairo. Discovered the trematode causing schistosomiasis. Died of typhus aged 37.

Blakemore, Arthur Hendley   80, 245
1897–1970. Assistant Professor of Surgery, Columbia University, New York.

Bordet, Jules   280
1870–1961. Bacteriologist, Institut Pasteur, Paris.

Bouin, Pol   137
1870–1962. Pioneer French histologist of Strasbourg.

Brodrick, Norman John Lee QC   19
Born 1912. Chairman of Departmental Committee on Death Certification and Coroners 1964.

Brook, Joseph   272, 274
Born 1915. Physician, St Paul's and University Hospitals, Saskatoon, Saskatchewan, Canada.

Brook, Morris H   272, 274
1911–1967. Surgeon to St Paul's and City Hospitals, Saskatoon, Canada.

Brook, Max   272, 274
Born 1920. A dental surgeon and brother of the above also contributed to the development of the Brook airway.

Bruce, Sir David   153
1855–1931. Graduated in Edinburgh. Joined the Army Medical Service. Discovered the cause of Malta fever, *Micrococcus melitensis*, later called *Brucella melitensis*.

Bunnell, Walls Willard   164, 168, 188
1902–1965. Member of the staff of Hartford Hospital, Hartford, Connecticut, USA. Co-discoverer of the Paul-Bunnell test for infectious mononucleosis.

Burnet, Sir (Frank) Macfarlane, OM FRS.   194
Born 1899. Professor of Experimental Medicine, University of Melbourne, Australia.

Casoni, Tomaso   117
1880–1933. Italian physician at Clinica Medica, Sassari, Sardinia.

Catterall, Mary   112
Born 1922. Consultant-in-charge Fast Neutron Clinic, MRC Cyclotron Unit, Royal Postgraduate Medical School, London. Previously lecturer in Clinical Physiology, Middlesex Hospital Medical School, London.

Celsius, Anders   59
1701–1744. Swedish physicist and astronomer. Invented the centigrade thermometer.

Cheyne, John   264
1777–1836. Graduated in Edinburgh in 1795. Physician to the Meath Hospital, Dublin. First Professor of Medicine at the Royal College of Physicians of Ireland.

Churchill, Sir Winston Spencer   83
1874–1965. British statesman. He led the British people in the Second World War. Prime Minister 1940–45, 1951–55. Honorary American citizen.

Conn, Jerome W.   144, 159
Born 1907. Head of the Department of Endocrinology, University of Michigan, Ann Arbor, Michigan, USA. Discovered primary aldosteronism.

Coombs, Robert Royston Amos, ScD, FRS   159
Born 1921. Quick Professor of Biology and Head of Immunology Division, University of Cambridge.

Cope, Constantin   89
Born 1927. Vascular radiologist, Albert Einstein Medical Center, Philadelphia, Pennsylvania, USA.

Coulter, Wallace
Born 1915. DSc Westminster College, Fulton, Missouri, USA. American Electronics engineer who discovered the modulation of an electric current path of small dimensions by the passage of individual particles through it and who made the first electronic blood cell counter.

Cushing, Harvey Williams   205, 206, 208, 212
1869–1939. Moseley Professor of Surgery, Harvard. Surgeon-in-Chief, Peter Bent Brigham Hospital, Boston, Maryland, USA.

Duchenne, Guillame Benjamin Armand   144

1806–1875. French neurologist; author of *Physiologie des Mouvements*.

Langdon-Down, John Langdon Haydon   8
1828–1896. Physician Superintendent, Normansfield, an institution for feeble-minded children. Assistant Physician to the London Hospital.

Ehrlich, Paul   75
1854–1915. German-Jewish bacteriologist, Serum Institute, Paul Ehrlich-strasse, Frankfurt-on-Main, Germany. Discovered salvarsan for the treatment of syphilis. Nobel prizewinner 1908.

Elisha,   271
The son of Shaphet of Abel-meholah of the tribe of Issachor. The chief prophet and holy man of Israel (*see* I Kings XIX).

Ellison, Edwin Homer   214
1918–1970. Professor of Surgery. Marquette University School of Medicine. Director of Surgery Milwaukee County Hospital.

Fahrenheit, Gabriel Daniel   59
1686–1736. German physicist who introduced the mercury thermometer about 1715.

Felix, Arthur   204
1887–1956. Born in Poland. Graduated in Vienna. Worked for the Hadassah Medical Organisation in Tel Aviv and at The Lister Institute in London. Director of the Central Reference Laboratory. Discovered, with Edmund Weil, the Weil–Felix test for typhus.

Foley, Frederic Eugene Basil   76
1891–1960. Urologist, St Paul, Minnesota, USA.

Fredrickson, Donald Sharp   221
Born 1924. Director of the National Institutes of Health, Bethesda, Maryland, USA.

Frei, Wilhelm Siegmund   117
1885–1943. German bacteriologist. Dermatologist, Berlin-Spandau Municipal Hospital and later at the Montefiore Hospital, New York.

Gram, Christian   249, 258
1853–1938. Physician-in-Chief, Royal Frederick's Hospital and Professor of Medicine, Copenhagen, Denmark.

Guillain, Georges   212
1876–1961. Neurologist of La Salpêtrière, Paris, France.

Guthrie, Robert   189
Born 1916. Professor of Pediatrics and Microbiology, State University of New York, Buffalo, New York.

Hagedorn, Werner H   116
1831–94. Surgeon in Magdeburg, Germany.

Handley, Anthony J.   262
Born 1942. Consultant Physician, Colchester District Hospitals, England.

Hartmann, Alexis Frank   256
1898–1964. Professor of Pediatrics, University of Washington, St Louis, Missouri, USA.

Hartnup   172
The name of the family showing hyper-aminoaciduria and neurological symptoms.

Hashimoto, Hakaru   227
1881–1934. Japanese surgeon and general practitioner, Ayama-gun, Mie Prefecture, Japan.

Heaf, Frederick Roland George   119
1894-1973. Professor of Tuberculosis, University of Wales.

Heinz, Robert   194
1865-1924. Professor of Pharmacology, Erlangen, Germany.

Homans, John   63
1877-1954. Professor of Clinical Surgery, Harvard University, USA.

Horner, Johann Friedrich   8
1831-86. Professor of Ophthalmology, Zürich, Switzerland.

Ingram, James Mayhew   78
Born 1921. Professor of Obstetrics and Gynaecology, University of South Florida, USA. (Argyle is the brand name of the manufacturer of his catheter.)

Ivy, Andrew Conway   158
1893-1978. Professor of Biochemistry, Roosevelt University, Chicago, USA.

Jones, Henry Bence   151
1813-1873. Physician to St George's Hospital, London. An early biochemist.

Joule, James Prescott   60, 275
1818-1889. English physicist who researched on electromagnetism and determined the mechanical equivalent of heat.

Kiesselbach, Wilhelm   250
1839-1902. Professor of Otology, University of Erlangen, Germany.

King, Earl J   143
1901-1962. Biochemist, Banting Institute, Toronto, Canada, and later Professor of Clinical Pathology, University of London, England (Hammersmith Hospital).

Koplik, Henry   67
1858-1927. Paediatrician, Mount Sinai and Jewish Maternity Hospitals, New York.

Kveim, Morten Ansgar   117
1892-1966. Dermatologist, Rikshospitalet, Oslo, Norway.

Langerhans, Paul   213
1847-1888. Research worker, Virchow's Laborotary, Berlin Pathological Intitute. Professor of Pathological Anatomy, Freiburg.

Lee, Roger Irving   158
1881-1965. Professor of Hygiene, Harvard University, Boston, USA.

Leishman, Sir William Boog   65
1865-1926. Professor of Pathology, Army Medical College, Netley. Director of Army Medical Services. Discovered the cause of kalar-azar (leishmaniasis).

Levin, Abraham Louis   215
1880-1940. Clinical Professor of Medicine, Louisiana State University, USA.

Little, James Lawrence   250
1836-1885. Professor of Surgery, University of Vermont, USA.

Magnuson, Paul Budd   57
1884-1968. Protessor of Surgery, Department of Bone and Joint Surgery, North Western University Medical School, Chicago, USA.

McArdle, Brian   177
Born 1911. Member of the External Staff of the Medical Research

Council at Guy's Hospital, London.

Maegraith, Brian Gilmore 64
Born 1907. Professor of Tropical Medicine, University of Liverpool.

Mantoux, Charles 118
1877–1947. Physician at Le Cannet, near Cannes, France.

Menghini, Giorgio 103
Born 1916. Chief of Medicine, 'Porte Sole' Medical Centre, Perugia, Italy.

Menière, Prosper 8
1799–1862. Physician-in-Chief, Imperial Institute for Deaf Mutes, Paris.

Münchausen, Baron Hieronymous Karl Friedrich von 57
1720–1797. A German-born Russian cavalry officer who told exaggerated stories of his adventures.

Neisser, Albert Ludwig Siegmund 134
Head of Breslau Clinic, Germany. Discoverer of gonococcus

Newton, Sir Isaac 60
1642–1727. Author of *Principia* and discoverer of gravity, the spectrum and inventor of the calculus.

Nightingale, Florence 46
1820–1910. English nurse and pioneer of hospital reform. Originated a nursing service in the Crimean War and was known as The Lady with the Lamp.

Occam (or Ockham), William of 5
1270 or 1300–1349. English philosopher of the Order of Franciscans who were violently opposed to the temporal power of the Pope. His maxim known as Occam's razor states that 'Entities are not to be multiplied without necessity' ('Entia praeter necessitatem non sunt multiplicanda').

Osler, Sir William, Bt 42, 59
1849–1919. Professor of Medicine successively at Montreal, Philadelphia, Baltimore and Oxford.

Paget, Sir James 143, 174
1814–1899. Surgeon to St Bartholomew's Hospital, London. Described osteitis deformans in 1877.

Parkinson, James 234
1755–1824. General Practitioner of Shoreditch, London. Author of 'An essay on the shaking palsy' 1817.

Parkinson, Sir John 10, 246
1885–1976. Physician to the Cardiac Department, The London Hospital and the National Heart Hospital.

Pascal, Blaise 108
1623–1662. French mathematician who invented a calculating machine. Later turned to religion.

Pasteur, Louis 98
1822–1895. French chemist. Director of Scientific studies, École Normale, Paris. He made fundamental discoveries about fermentation.

Paul, John Rodman 164, 168, 188
1893–1971. Professor of Epidemiology and Preventive Medicine at Yale University, USA.

Queckenstedt, Hans Heinrich 126
1876–1918. Physician-in-Chief, City Hospital, Harburg near Hamburg, Germany. Described a test for determining the patency of the subarachnoid space. Killed in a street accident in 1918.

Ricketts, Howard Taylor 204
1871-1910. Professor of Pathology in the University of Pennsylvania.

Robertson, Douglas Moray Cooper Lamb Argyll 8
1837-1909. Ophthalmic Surgeon to the Royal Infirmary, Edinburgh. A great golfer, he won the gold medal of the Royal and Ancient Club of St Andrew's five times.

Rose, Harry M. 178, 195
Born 1906. Associate Professor of Microbiology, Columbia University, New York. Physician to the Prestbyterian Hospital, New York. (Rose discovered his test for rheumatoid disease in 1948 but, unknown to him, it had been discovered by Waaler in 1940. The test is known in Scandinavia as the Waaler-Rose test.)

Ryle, John 81, 138, 215
1899-1950. Physician to Guy's Hospital, London. Regius Professor of Physics at Cambridge and later of Social Medicine at Oxford.

Salmon, Brian Lawson 46
Born 1917. Chairman of the Committee on Senior Nursing Staff Structure. Chairman of the Camden and Islington Health Authority.

Salmon, Daniel Elmer 268
1850-1914. American veterinary pathologist. Practised at Newark, New Jersey. Later Head of the Veterinary Department, University of Montevideo, Uraguay.

Schilling, Robert Frederick 223
Born 1919. Professor of Medicine, University of Wisconsin Medical School, Madison, Wisconsin, USA.

Sengstaken, Robert William 80, 245
1923-1978. American neurosurgeon, Community Hospital, Glen Cove, New York.

Señorans, Juan B 79, 99
1859-1933. Professor of Toxicology, University of Buenos Aires, Argentina.

Silverman, Irving 122
Born 1904. Medical and surgical practitioner, Brooklyn, New York.

Simmonds, Morris 213
1858-1925. German general practitioner. Also Pathologist, Hospital of St George, Hamburg.

Sjögren, Henrik 173
Born 1889. Ophthalmologist; Lecturer in Rosengren Clinic, Gothenburg, Sweden.

Somogyi, Michael 148
1883-1971. Biochemist, St Louis, USA. Born in Austria-Hungary.

Stokes, William 264, 276
1804-1878. Graduated at Edinburgh in 1825. Physician to the Meath Hospital, Dublin. Regius Professor of Physic, Royal College of Surgeons of Ireland.

Thudichum, Ludwig Johann Wilhelm 250
1829-1901. A graduate of the University of Geissen, Germany, who settled in London in 1853 and became lecturer in pathological chemistry at St Thomas's Hospital. In later life he became interested in diseases of the nose.

Trendelenburg, Friedrich 84
1844-1924. Surgeon to the Friedrichshain Hospital, Berlin, and Professor of Surgery successively at Rostock, Bonn and Leipzig.

Treves, Sir Frederick 45
1853–1923. Surgeon to the London Hospital. Sergeant-surgeon to Queen Victoria, Edward VII and George V.

Trousseau, Armand xv
1801–1867. Physician to the Hôtel Dieu, Paris. Member of l'Académie de Médicine.

Tuffier, Marin Theodor 124
1857–1922. Surgeon to the Hopital de la Cité du Midi and the British Hertford Hospital, Paris.

Tunbridge, Sir Ronald Ernest O.B.E. 252
Born 1906. Professor of Medicine, University of Leeds. Consultant Physician, The General Infirmary at Leeds.

Turner-Warwick, Margaret Elizabeth Harvey 102
Born 1924. Professor of Medicine (Thoracicic Medicine), Cardio-Thoracic Institute, Brompton Hospital, London.

Valsalva, Antonio Maria 84
1666–1723. Professor of Anatomy, Bologna, Italy. Surgeon to the Hospital for Incurables, Bologna.

Venturi, Giovanni Battista 111
1746–1822. Professor of Physics, University of Pavia, Italy.

Waaler, Eric 178, 195
Born 1903. Professor of Pathology and Rector, University of Bergen, Norway.

Wassermann, August von 6
1866–1925. Director of the Kaiser Wilhelm Institute of Experimental Therapeutics, Berlin.

Weed, Lawrence Leonard 5
Born 1923. Microbiologist. Professor of Medicine and Community Medicine, University of Vermont, USA.

Weil, Edmund 204
1879–1922. Prague bacteriologist.

Wernicke, Carl 260
1848–1905. Professor of Psychiatry and Neurology in Breslau, Germany.

Westergren, Alf Wilhelm 165
1891–1968. Chief Physician, St Goran's Hospital, Stockholm and Professor at the Karolinska Institute.

White, Paul Dudley 158, 246
1886–1973. Eminent American cardiologist. Professor of Medicine at Harvard.

Widal, Georges Fernand Isidore 137, 165
1862–1929. Professor of Internal Medicine and later of Clinical Medicine, Paris. The inventor of sero-diagnosis.

Wilson, Samuel Alexander Kinnier 159, 204
1878–1937. Physician to the National Hospital for the Paralysed and Epileptic (later The National Hospital, Queen Square), London.

Wolff, Louis 246
1898–1972. A clinical professor of Medicine Emeritus at Harvard Medical School. Visiting physician at Beth Israel Hospital.

Wright, Basil Morton 109
Born 1912. Bioengineering Division, Clinical Research Centre, Harrow, Middlesex.

Zollinger, Robert Milton 214
Born 1903. Emeritus Professor of Surgery, Ohio State University, USA. Editor of *The American Journal of Surgery*.

Index